# the
# HORMONE
# MYTH

## HOW JUNK SCIENCE,
## GENDER POLITICS & LIES ABOUT PMS
## KEEP WOMEN DOWN

### ROBYN STEIN DELUCA, PhD

New Harbinger Publications, Inc.

## Publisher's Note

*This publication is designed to provide accurate and authoritative information in regard to the subject matter covered. It is sold with the understanding that the publisher is not engaged in rendering psychological, financial, legal, or other professional services. If expert assistance or counseling is needed, the services of a competent professional should be sought.*

Distributed in Canada by Raincoast Books

Copyright © 2017 by Robyn Stein DeLuca
New Harbinger Publications, Inc.
5674 Shattuck Avenue
Oakland, CA 94609
www.newharbinger.com

Cover design by Amy Shoup

Edited by Jennifer Holder

Indexed by James Minkin

All Rights Reserved

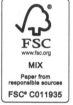 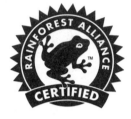

### Library of Congress Cataloging-in-Publication Data

Names: DeLuca, Robyn Stein, author.
Title: The hormone myth : how junk science, gender politics, and lies about PMS keep women down / Robyn Stein DeLuca.
Description: Oakland, CA : New Harbinger Publications, 2017. | Includes bibliographical references.
Identifiers: LCCN 2016050783 (print) | LCCN 2017020425 (ebook) | ISBN 9781626255104 (PDF e-book) | ISBN 9781626255111 (ePub) | ISBN 9781626255098 (pbk)
Subjects: LCSH: Women--Psychology. | Women--Mental health. | Hormones. | BISAC: HEALTH & FITNESS / Women's Health. | SOCIAL SCIENCE / Women's Studies. | MEDICAL / Gynecology & Obstetrics. | SELF-HELP / Personal Growth / General.
Classification: LCC HQ1206 (ebook) | LCC HQ1206 .D3627 2017 (print) | DDC 155.3/33--dc23
LC record available at https://lccn.loc.gov/2016050783

19    18    17

10    9    8    7    6    5    4    3    2    1          First Printing

"*The Hormone Myth* is a bracing, accurate breath of fresh air. It turns conventional wisdom about hormones on its head, and provides a far more liberating view of women's health than what we've all been taught."

—**Christiane Northrup, MD**, OB/GYN physician and author of the *New York Times* bestsellers *Goddesses Never Age*; *Women's Bodies, Women's Wisdom*; and *The Wisdom of Menopause*

"This is a book for every woman who has ever been asked 'Are you on the rag?' after she voices an unpopular opinion or expresses an 'unfeminine' emotion. Read it, share it with your friends, and join the movement to bust the hormone myth once and for all."

—**Joan C. Chrisler, PhD**, editor of *Women's Reproductive Health*

"This eye-opening book covers female developmental milestones (e.g., menarche, pregnancy, menopause) where the 'hormone myth' is characterized by an excessive focus on biology over modifiable environmental factors, while ignoring empirical findings in favor of pseudoscience, sensationalism, scaremongering, and the fragilization of women. One chapter at a time, from Aristotle to Trump, the author weaves together historical, cultural, and economic developments that—intentionally or not—create and maintain this hormone myth. The author argues cogently that the eventual impact on women is a net negative: despite a few short-term social gains, these myths keep women feeling, and being perceived, as overly emotional and less suitable for competent leadership. This is a must-read for any person who wants to know what science can truly tell us about the relationship of hormones to women's mental health, and how to help debunk entrenched societal myths that perpetuate gender inequities at home and work."

—**Jacqueline Pistorello, PhD**, research faculty at Counseling Services at University of Nevada, Reno, and coauthor of *Finding Life Beyond Trauma*

"*The Hormone Myth* not only helps women recognize the cultural forces boxing them in, but provides the tools needed to be smart consumers of some of the scientific research that falsely insinuates they are 'hormonal maniacs.' DeLuca brinoice to the stubborn myth of women's emotic

—**Susan Pincus, MD**, family physician

For my daughters, Caroline and Jamie

# Contents

# The Myth That Traps Us

"Women's hormones make them crazy." Everyone knows this. The ups and downs of our monthly hormone cycle turn women into moody, irrational, angry, unpleasant, PMSing witches. Pregnancy makes us incapable and incoherent. After childbirth, dangerous changes in hormones can cause postpartum depression so severe we can harm ourselves or our babies. And then as menopause approaches, comes, and goes, we get despondent, depressed, and crazy as loons. Therefore, women are to be feared, kept under wraps, and put in their place not just by men but by humanity as a whole.

We've all heard PMS jokes, coddled a pregnant woman, followed horrifying accounts of postpartum murder in the news, and seen a sitcom character come unhinged because she is "of that age." I'm sure you and many women you know have had your anger explained away because it's "your time of the month," had sadness you felt in the weeks after childbirth chalked up to "just hormones," or found your new aspirations in life dismissed because you are just being "menopausal" and not yourself.

Everyone agrees that changing hormones make women nuts; it's a fact of life we all unfortunately have to live with. Right?

Wrong. Hormones don't make women crazy.

How can that be? How can something so taken for granted actually be wildly overstated? This persistent and willful ignorance of the truth is what makes the hormone myth so dangerous. Women individually and as a whole, all men who care about us, families, marriages, businesses, communities, politics—the very structures of our societies—are harmed by believing it.

Because what everyone "knows" is actually inaccurate. A large body of scientific research says that fluctuating reproductive hormones *don't* play a major role in women's mental health, because when women's emotional stability is measured by the frequency and severity of mood swings they experience over time, it is in fact similar to the stability of men.

Surprised? Well, here's the kicker: psychologists have known that since the early 1990s but it is probably news to you. This shows the power of the hormone myth's spell over us and speaks volumes about all the profiting, political-maneuvering, salary- and career-repressing, and relationship-appeasing motives that compel us to keep believing in and perpetuating something that's just not true for every woman.

Yes, some women suffer disturbing physical symptoms because of hormone change. There are women who have terrible cramps during their periods and perimenopausal women can have twenty hot flashes a day— their complaints are definitely real and may need medical attention. And there are some women who do experience distressing emotional symptoms associated with hormone change that require treatment. But they are a minority. The hormone myth says that *all* women become emotionally erratic when their hormones fluctuate and that is simply not true. Mistakenly attributing any negative emotion women have to hormones comes with many costs, and I wrote this book because I believe we will all be better off once we stop blaming women's feelings on their hormones.

I use the term "myth" to describe a belief that is based on faulty information or reasoning, but has been accepted by society and serves, in some way, to maintain the status quo. The power of these myths is wide-reaching, long-lasting, and seemingly intractable. The hormone myth is built on the foundation of the ancient but persistent idea that women are inferior to men because of a biological-based emotionality and on evidence from poorly done scientific studies conducted in the mid-twentieth century. The myth has been perpetuated through all types of media, whether on television, at news outlets, in books and magazines, or throughout the Internet. And as you'll see, many parties benefit financially and socially from the maintenance of the hormone myth—even as it causes women's health, professional advancement, and personal relationships to suffer.

Here are some important truths that psychologists have known since the early 1990s. The majority of studies used to support the existence of PMS were deeply flawed and unreliable; high-quality studies of women's emotions during the menstrual cycle show no evidence of a widespread "syndrome." There is also no evidence that pregnancy affects cognitive skills and memory. It is clear that, while many variables contribute to postpartum depression, changing hormones isn't one of them. And despite the fact that older women are widely represented as sexless, depressed, and deranged, studies consistently find that the majority of menopause-aged women feel happy and satisfied with their lives.

Psychologists and physicians also know that some women have symptoms related to reproductive events. It's common for menstruating women to deal with backaches, cramping, and occasional irritability. Pregnant women's hormones do increase dramatically. In the first few days after childbirth, weepiness and mood swings frequently do occur. And hot flashes are the most common symptom of perimenopause.

But the evidence is clear: for the great majority of women, changes in hormones caused by reproductive events don't cause mental disorders.

Many people resist the idea that this myth is false. And why wouldn't they, it's so ingrained. The idea that a woman's reproductive system is responsible for her emotional state has been around since the time of the ancient Greeks. Hippocrates theorized that the womb wandered within the body, so when it landed next to the brain, unusual emotions and behaviors resulted. Aristotle, arguably the most influential thinker of Western civilization, viewed women as psychologically and emotionally inferior to men because of the biological deficiencies he saw in women. He famously referred to a female as "a deformed male" and said that "[w]e must look upon the female character as being a sort of natural deficiency." This view permeated Western thought for a millenium.[1] In the mid-1200s, philosopher Thomas Aquinas reiterated Aristotle's views, when he wrote that "[w]oman is defective and misbegotten" and concluded that a woman should be subject to a man because the male biological makeup provides a superior capacity for reason.[2] Christian scholars in Europe also weighed in on the biological basis of women's weaknesses, and in 1487 published and widely distributed a manual for witch hunters called *The Hammer of Witches*. In it, they explained that women were more likely than men to be tempted by Satan because they were "more concerned with things of the flesh" and "feebler both in mind and body."[3]

Physicians of the 1800s understood that in women's bodies, the brain and reproductive organs were connected, so when they fell out of sync, hysteria resulted. They defined it as feelings of "anxiety, irritability, and nervousness."[4] In the 1940s and 50s, doctors introduced the idea that women's reproductive hormones caused them physical and emotional upheaval. For decades they warned women that if they didn't replace their "lost" hormones, they would lose both their beauty and their agreeable nature. The uterus continued to be under suspicion as well, and into the 1970s hysterectomies were thought to be appropriate for treating women with excessive anxiety.[5]

The persistent and repeated messages over the millennia that women's reproductive organs cause mental instability and that this biology by nature makes them inferior to men in their thinking has solidified the concept of women as substandard humans, in contrast to the ideal rational male. This has been used to keep women in their secondary places at home, at work, and in all elements of society.

Today, messages about women being at the mercy of their reproductive biology continue on in popular culture and the media. Newspapers and books need to be sold and websites need traffic, so the more sensational the better. Audiences find "essential differences" between men and women fascinating, and become glued to stories of the crazed women who make headlines. When these audiences hear scientific studies reported that support their assumptions, they accept them and opinions are bolstered. However, when people hear evidence that contrasts their beliefs, they are more likely to write it off as inaccurate or an outlier. These biases unfortunately emphasize popular studies—no matter what quality methods were used or how rigged they were for certain results—that show gender differences over those that find no differences. Because, while more psychological and medical research indicate greater similarities than differences, people find it easier to accept the cultural message that women are biologically motivated, emotional, and unreliable, and men are rational, logical, and steady. Because it is something they already believe.

The underlying question here is, if there is so little fact to support the hormone myth, why does it persist? The answer is vast and involves many parties who are invested financially, ideologically, and emotionally in maintaining it. Examples include pharmaceutical companies that reap enormous profits by convincing a healthy woman that she needs daily medication. Physicians who prescribe daily hormones benefit financially by the many visits required to monitor a woman's health. When psychologists have an official diagnosis, they receive insurance reimbursement for treating her. A husband has a way to deflect his wife's anger away from him with a joke and she has something to blame when life doesn't feel right. Politicians and religious leaders have fuel for promoting traditional gender roles and the limitations that come with them. Whatever the motivation is for continuing, and even exacerbating, the hormone myth, it succeeds in keeping a woman in line and in her place by preventing anyone from trusting her mental state—especially herself.

Remarkably, women hesitate to even consider evidence that hormones don't rule their lives. Yes, the myth is a cultural tidal wave in an ocean of history and it's really hard not to internalize a message so forcefully pushed at you. The result is that women have difficulty doubting it, much less resisting it. And it's also true that women do benefit from the idea that moments of anger or irritability are out of their control. It allows them to maintain the feminine ideal of constant availability and pleasantness by giving them an acceptable pressure valve they can occasionally release steam through. Hormones can explain away an error in judgment, a mistake, an insulting slip, or a harsh tone. But these limited benefits come with many costs.

As you will read about in the chapters that follow, the hormone myth encourages stereotypes of women as irrational—which dismisses and discounts us. It contributes to the dangerous idea that women's normal biological processes are sicknesses that require treatment—resulting in excessive, expensive, and sometimes harmful "cures." It perpetuates clichés like the good woman who always puts the needs of others first, the elderly lady who feels sad and purposeless, the menopausal boss who takes it out on her assistant, the unpredictable mother whose moods are impossible to navigate—all of which box us into other people's assumptions. There are many consequences to women's tendency to attribute their anger to raging hormones, including not dealing with the real issues that are causing their emotional upset and not looking to their emotions for vital self-knowledge. Ultimately, the hormone myth makes it harder for women to feel confident, express themselves in relationships, and conduct their lives with honesty and accountability.

It's not easy to resist thousands of years of mythology, but it can be done. There are ways to recognize and even abandon this false vision of women, and I will share them in the pages to come. If we can overcome all the bad science, hype, and blame games—personally and culturally—the benefits are huge. As fewer people buy into the hormone myth, perceptions of women's abilities and mental health can become much closer to reality. This allows women to be judged on their own merits rather than folklore, which consequently expands educational and professional opportunities. Women who take ownership of their emotions gain the power to understand and address conditions that make them unhappy. And mothers can ultimately stop the myth in its tracks by modeling a positive attitude about reproductive functions and inspiring children to develop healthy skepticism about the ways women in all cycles and stages of life are portrayed in the media.

This hormone myth keeps women down through a complex snarl of storylines that we need to take apart and analyze. My hope is that by untangling them and giving them a lucid stare we will be able to see the players more clearly—with all their motivations and influences—and get closer to the truth about women: that most of us are very high functioning the great majority of the time. We need to first step out of the myth so we can step into reality.

# CHAPTER 1

# Meet the Menstrual Monster and the PMSing Bitch

"You're a woman now." That's what girls hear when they get their first period. With this event marking such a momentous leap toward womanhood, we have to wonder: what does menstruation mean about being a woman?

Girls learn about it from many sources in addition to their mother, sisters, or a grandmother. Booklets provided by tampon and pad companies are often used in elementary school health classes that focus on negative aspects of menstruation, warning girls about cramps, moodiness, and leaks. Websites run by these companies[1] and also organizations that focus on girls' health[2] share, as a matter of fact, that hormones can wreak havoc with your moods. Books marketed to girls about puberty like American Girls' *The Care and Keeping of You 2: The Body Book for Older Girls* also warn them about how the menstrual cycle is an "emotional rollercoaster."[3] And of course, there are a multitude of jokes about menstruation told at home and at school that portray menstruating women as violent, irrational, and out of control.[4]

When girls hear "You're a woman now," they also hear that this essential part of being a woman sucks.

When the media uses phrases like "the cycle of misery," "a hormonal rollercoaster," or "the monthly monster" to describe menstruation, young girls can't miss the idea that menstruation is a hormonally fueled disaster bearing down on them.[5] It's so gross and shameful that code words are needed to simply speak about it, like "my friend is here," "it's that time of the month," or "I'm on the rag." When I was a teenager, ads for tampons featured women in flowing, white dresses on the beach who vaguely mentioned "nature" or "that time." Despite the euphemisms, I remember wanting to crawl behind the living-room couch when my father was there and these commercials came on. Fathers and daughters definitely didn't talk about periods or tampons, and for the most part that remains true today.[6]

Both men and women have seriously negative impressions of menstruating women. College students describe them as "sad," "moody," "tired," "weak," "desperate," "whining," "unpredictable," "incapable," and "less likeable."[7] Many people also see menstruating women as less competent.[8] So, as girls approach the beginning of menstruation, they join the multitude of people who think menstruation is awful and that menstruating women are awful. This attitude initiates them into the hormone myth and many girls experience menarche, the beginning of menstruation, as "unwanted," "polluting," and as a "form of invasion."[9]

Psychologists have identified the many ways menstruation is stigmatized and the harm that stigmatization brings.[10] When a girl begins to menstruate, she is stigmatized by her reproductive potential. Parents may restrict her freedom, telegraphing messages that her maturing body is something dangerous that can get her in trouble. Also, menstrual blood is commonly seen as viscerally disgusting. In 2015, a woman posted a picture on Instagram that showed a menstrual leak on her sweatpants. Instagram quickly removed it, stating that it was not within the website's guidelines, which prohibit photos that are not "appropriate for a diverse audience." Women go to great lengths to prevent leaks because of the social humiliation they can bring. Menstrual products are designed and advertised to maintain secrecy, implying that menstruation is so awful tampons and pads need to be tiny so they can be carried discreetly.

Could the "Welcome to womanhood" sign be painted any uglier?

## A POPULAR ACCUSATION

Accusing someone of "being on the rag" conveys how contemptible menstruation is to us. If a woman complains about something to her boyfriend and he responds, not by addressing the issue, but by asking "Is it that time of the month?", he's saying that she's being irrationally irritable. He's making it clear that she would have to be out of her mind to be upset by such a thing. Because the operating assumption is that women on their periods are, basically, out of their minds.

Even women hurl the menstrual accusation at other women or at themselves. Despite the fact that the great majority of women are high functioning throughout their menstrual cycle, and even though the accusation might draw on evidence contradictory to their own experience, still women say, "Don't worry about it, you're just PMSing" or "I don't make major decisions when I'm on my period." So why buy into this part of the hormone myth? It may reflect the depth of women's internalization,[11] as the ubiquitous idea that menstruation makes women crazy becomes tough to resist in all our relationships. One twin I know used to say about the other, "Most women are grumpy one week a month—my sister is only nice one week a month, because she has PMS, DMS, and AMS: pre, during, and after menstrual syndrome." In general, people tend to think they are better than others, so it's also possible that women with few menstrual-related symptoms convince themselves that they don't have these kinds of troubles because they are better able to control themselves than most women.[12]

Some say the most devastating use of the menstrual accusation is from man to man. When one man asks another "Is it that time of the month?," the result is total emasculation. The menstrual accusation accomplishes this by first making fun of a man for expressing emotions that are considered to be typically feminine and therefore weak. It then denigrates a man because it evokes the male taboo against doing anything "like a girl." It condemns him for being like a woman in the worst possible way.[13]

In all its uses, the menstruation accusation effectively invalidates someone's emotions or opinions by making menstruation synonymous with moodiness and unreasonability.

## DOES MENSTRUATION TRULY KEEP US FROM FUNCTIONING WELL?

The idea that the menstrual cycle causes women to have problems functioning is one that has captivated psychologists for a long time. As early as 1914, one of the few female psychologists at the time, Leta Hollingworth, studied the relationship between the phases of the menstrual cycle and women's intellectual and sensory-motor skills. She found no relationship.

In the 1970s and 80s, numerous studies were conducted on the potential impact of the menstrual cycle on a wide variety of skills including spelling, writing, memory, academic performance, arithmetic, spatial tasks, factory performance, judgment, and social skills such as detecting others' moods from facial expressions. The research overwhelmingly showed that the phases of menstruation had no impact on any of these skills, and a few studies in the 1990s and 2000s even showed improved performance during menstruation.[14]

Recent studies of these variables, using more sophisticated methodology, continue to find no support for any causal relationship between menstrual phase and cognitive functions.[15] But these studies seldom get press coverage. The rare studies that have found an impact get enormous attention in newspapers, television, and online, trumpeting the "convincing" evidence that women's bodies really do make them crazy.[16]

## WE'VE ALL LEARNED THESE ATTITUDES AND THEY HURT US MONTHLY

In Elizabeth Wurtzel's memoir *Prozac Nation*, she recounts her mother's response to her first period: "Oh hell, your period. This is where the trouble starts." When a mother reacts to her daughter's menstruation with negativity, the ramifications are powerful and long-lasting. In response to menarche, some parents restrict their daughters' freedoms and make it clear that their physical development is dangerous.[17] Their growing up is not good in the way it used to be, when a new notch on the doorway growth-chart was an important and positive thing. When one of my daughters was becoming quite curvy, we heard that my husband "better get a shotgun" more than once, a comment that reduced her down to a desirable thing that we owned and better protect. Nobody suggests getting a shotgun to protect a fourteen-year-old boy going through a growth spurt. Instead, the physical development of boys is greeted with positivity and admiration with comments like "The girls are gonna go crazy for him!"

Expectations are powerful predictors of experience; women taught negative attitudes about menstruation when young are more likely to report disturbing physical symptoms related to the menstrual cycle.[18] Just as the well-known placebo effect is powerful, so is the lesser-known "nocebo effect." This occurs when the expectation of symptoms increases the likelihood of experiencing the symptoms.[19] One study on the effectiveness of aspirin illustrates how an emphasis on negative possible outcomes can influence the experience of symptoms. People were recruited for the study from several different locations. However, the consent form that participants read and signed was slightly different depending on location: some locations included information about possible gastrointestinal side effects of aspirin and some locations didn't. The people who did receive that information were *six times* more likely to withdraw from the study because of gastrointestinal side effects compared to the people who did not receive that warning.[20]

And this was after just one instance of receiving a single negative message. Girls get negative messages about menstruation continuously and from many different sources. What if a mother responds to her daughter's arguing back by saying "What's wrong with you? Is it your period?" Or if a girl who drops a tampon at school gets taunted as a "bleeder"? Or if a commercial assures her that a pad is so thin, no one will ever know she has her period? This unrelenting stream of negativity has a cumulative effect on how a girl views her body and how she experiences it.

When we raise girls to expect substantial physical and emotional symptoms prior to menstruation, we increase the likelihood they will experience them. People tend to ignore symptoms they don't expect and pay attention to those they do.[21] Research tells us that the more women believe that everyone gets PMS, the more likely they are to erroneously report that they have it. When asked if they had PMS, many women said "yes," but after providing two months of daily logs of mood and other symptoms, no relationship was found between their psychological symptoms and the time of the month.[22]

## POP ATTITUDES HURT US PERMANENTLY

Learning these stigmatizing messages about menstruation can impact women's future health, sexuality, and self-esteem.[23] Based on a review of relevant research, psychologists suggest that negative attitudes about menstruation are related to the objectification that women routinely experience. Western culture portrays the female body as something to be gazed upon for the pleasure of others. Women internalize this objectification and respond to it by monitoring their bodies so they are always attractive and acceptable. We check our makeup before leaving the house, do what we can to have a good hair day, and devote a lot of effort to choosing flattering clothes. There is strong evidence that women who self-objectify have especially shameful attitudes about menstruation and reproductive processes in general. They are more likely to use birth control that will suppress menstruation for months at a time—a practice for which the health consequences are not yet fully understood.[24]

Attitudes about menstruation also appear to impact women's overall feelings of health and self-image. Many women spend a lot of time thinking about what they perceive to be their body's flaws and trying to figure out ways to change them or mask them. Who hasn't tried diet pills, liquid diets, or the latest exercise fad? One study of women's attitudes about menstruation found that women who report having positive attitudes about it are also more likely to report feeling physically fit, illness-free, and satisfied with their bodies compared to women with negative menstrual attitudes.[25] Focusing on health and fitness is one thing, but all the time and energy we spend trying to get our bodies to fit an unrealistic ideal could be better invested in work, relationships, and enjoying life.

These attitudes also have an impact on a woman's sexual activity and satisfaction. Sexuality is an important element of the human experience—it creates a wonderful high, deep intimate emotional connection, and intense physical pleasure. Women with positive attitudes about their periods report a higher level of comfort with their sexuality.[26] On the other hand, women who feel shameful about menstruation participate in more sexual risk-taking behavior, like having sex without condoms, than women who are comfortable with menstruation, which threatens their physical health and well-being.[27]

Conceptualizing menstruation as a nasty, crazy-making thing also threatens women's professional advancement. Even though women have made great career advances in the past fifty years, they still make up a miniscule number of those with the most power in American industry and government. Women account for a paltry 4 percent of the CEOs of Fortune 500 companies[28] which makes their anemic—but all-time high—hold on 20 percent of the seats in Congress seem impressive. The myth of the menstrual monster is to blame for some of this. When people think that menstruation affects women's abilities to be rational, competent beings, it is easier to justify limiting their access to powerful positions. During Senate hearings on the confirmation of Supreme Court Justice Sonia Sotomayor, conservative commentator G. Gordon Liddy focused not on her education or judicial experience, but on the debilitating effect he thought menstruation would have on her judgment: "Let's hope that the key conferences aren't when she's menstruating or something, or just before she's going to menstruate. That would really be bad. Lord knows what we would get then."[29]

In our hormone-myth culture, if you want to prevent a woman from taking a powerful position, you don't need to criticize her experience, skills, or politics. All you have to do is pull the "crazy period" card and you've invoked suspicion about her ability to be a rational human being. In the first Republican presidential primary debate for the 2016 election, Fox News anchor Megyn Kelly aggressively questioned Donald Trump. To discredit her, he later tweeted that she was a "bimbo," "not very professional," and that "[y]ou could see there was blood coming out of her eyes, blood coming out of her wherever." It was the menstruation accusation heard round the world and, while the response from social and mainstream media was critical,[30] it's worth noting that this episode did not cause any decrease in Trump's poll numbers at the time, nor keep him from being elected president.

One policy that illustrates the conflicted status of menstruation in the workplace is menstrual leave. In recent years, employers in England and Asian countries like South Korea, China, and Indonesia, instituted a policy in which female workers had specifically allotted, paid days off for when their periods became too much to bear. On one hand, some feminists saw this as a positive thing: menstruation is being acknowledged and the women who have a hard time can care for themselves without losing pay. But many feminists objected because it buys into the idea that *all* women are crippled by their periods and are therefore rendered unqualified and incompetent every month—when the truth is that most women are not.[31]

## ALL WOMEN GET PMS, RIGHT?

Everyone thinks that all women get PMS because that's what we hear from virtually every source of information in America. The "fact" of widespread PMS is declared in medical websites and books, magazines and newspapers, television shows and movies, and social media and in-person conversation. All of these sources convey that if you don't assume all women get PMS, you're the crazy one. But as you'll see in chapter 2, there is no scientific reason to believe all women turn into deranged she-devils due to menstrual cycling.

When you take a look at all this talk, several consistent themes emerge: that PMS is a known fact; that it turns women into crazed bitches who will hurt you; and that PMS is a card that can be pulled to get out of jail, free. I'll discuss each theme in depth so you can more clearly perceive the hold that the hormone myth has on us.

## PMS Is a Known Fact

In American media, there is no debate about whether women suffer from PMS or not. Widely respected newspapers have run stories describing it as a known, common affliction. In various articles in recent years, the *New York Times* has stated that anywhere between 50 to 80 percent of women suffer from PMS to the degree that it impairs their daily lives and relationships.[32] The *Wall Street Journal* has noted that "many women suffer from PMS."[33] A few news websites like the *Huffington Post* and *Jezebel* have run stories exploring the possibility that PMS does not affect great swaths of women, but articles like this are drips in the firehose of information, coming few and far between.

The most popular television medical personality, Dr. Mehmet Oz, also is a firm believer in widespread PMS. His shows and website have promoted PMS treatments and "attack plans."[34] To bolster the case that PMS afflicts most women, Dr. Oz's website claims that 85 percent of women have at least one symptom of PMS. Does anyone imagine that having only one symptom of lung cancer—say, a cough—is in any way indicative of having lung cancer? Of course not. We don't need a medical degree to understand that just *one* symptom of a disease has absolutely no diagnostic meaning.

Reputable websites for medical information like WebMD present PMS as an extremely commonly experienced, verified psychological disorder caused by hormones[35]—even here, the cultural zeitgeist trumps known science. A quick Google search will bring up a cornucopia of PMS treatments, workshops, and clinics. One doctor's website claims that 30 to 40 percent of women suffer from PMS symptoms that impair their daily functioning.[36] If this were true, it would mean that a third of all women consistently function in a highly compromised way. That's unlikely.

Books about PMS abound. A visit to the local bookstore and a search on Amazon.com result in a multitude of books on treating it. One with a title that promises *30 Days to No More PMS* warns readers that between 40 and 60 percent of all women currently suffer from PMS or are destined to. That book, as well as *The Bible Cure for PMS and Mood Swings* describe PMS symptoms as lasting as long as fourteen days of every month. That's half of life! How can we possibly think that such a large percentage of women are so incapacitated? And according to the *The Bible Cure*, PMS symptoms include irritability, decreased sex drive, headache, breast pain, abdominal bloating, stress and tension, fatigue, mood swings, depression, backache, and swelling in the feet, ankles, and fingers. All at once? If anyone has all those symptoms at the same time, they need to get to the hospital because there is something seriously wrong.

You don't even have to be a woman to have a PMS book written for you—there are books for men like *PMS: A Guy's Roadmap (In Case You Won't Ask for Directions.): The Secrets to Living with a Lady's Cycle* with a title that says it all, and *The Prince and the PMS* which claims to give "men the tools they need to walk an estrogen-slick tightrope once a month without losing their minds, tempers, or sense of humor."

Popular women's magazines regularly run stories about PMS, with titles that show the editors of these magazines assume that everyone knows what PMS is, and that most women suffer from it. Here are some examples of articles run in 2016.[37]

*Shape:* "The Best Way to Reduce Your PMS Symptoms, According to Science"

*Glamour:* "What to Eat to Make Your Period Suck Less"

*Self:* "8 Habits That Are Making Your Period Even Worse"

*Good Housekeeping:* "7 Natural Period Remedies That Actually Work"

*Cosmopolitan:* "19 SUPER-Real Period Things All Dudes Need to Understand"

These headlines reveal the bias toward experiencing it as something to work to ward off, as if your life depended on it. It is universally understood as awful, and that women have a responsibility to "beat it."

Popular television shows often show female characters PMSing. In an episode of *The Big Bang Theory*, Penny has eaten all of her Halloween chocolate and comes home with another big bag of candy and says to Sheldon and Leonard, "It's a rough month when Halloween and PMS hit at the same time," and they smile in understanding.[38] On *The New Girl*, Zooey Deschanel's character announces her PMS to her male roommates as a regularly occurring phenomenon and suggests it might make her "kick the testicles clean off" them.[39] Which leads to the next recurring myth about PMS I want to discuss.

## PMS Turns Women into Crazed Bitches Who Will Hurt You

Just as everyone knows that most women get PMS, they also know that it causes a nasty insanity that makes life hellish for all. Both male and female comedians have deeply plumbed the trope of the PMSing woman as a dangerous psychopath. I could easily fill twenty pages with these kinds of jokes; here are just a few.[40]

"I have PMS and GPS, which means I'm a bitch and I will find you."

"I have PMS. Be afraid. Be very afraid."

"You earned a gold star! You had PMS and didn't kill anyone."

The most memorable joke I've ever heard came from my daughter's biology teacher. He described PMS as "Poor Man Syndrome," and the sounds of me screaming when I heard that are still reverberating around the universe. I could go on and on and I'm sure you could recite a few of your own.

The legendary premenstrual monster is well-documented on Twitter. In an analysis of one week of English-language tweets, researchers found that premenstrual women were characterizing themselves as:

Having insatiable cravings: "Ate fries and chocolate for breakfast… this PMS is strong today."

Being unable to control reactions to various irritants: "I'm at the point in my PMS where even old people in love are bumming me out."

Reacting to notably insensitive male behavior: "I told my boyfriend I was PMSing and he nodded so I stabbed him."[41]

Also, the general theme of malfunction was applied to many different subjects, with tweets like "Hmmm, God's not listening?? Maybe it's Her time of the month," and once when Twitter was not working efficiently, a tweeter accused it of "PMSing."

Men's disdain for women with PMS is reflected in recent tweets like "Why do they call it PMS? Because mad cow disease was taken," and in the hashtags #Liesbitchestell and #Womendoshitlike. Just like the menstruation accusation, the suggestion of a man PMSing is meant to be the most degrading. A recent tweet about pop-star Justin Bieber said, "@ justinbieber is having a pms moment...anyone have a tampon?" It was meant to put him down in the most emasculating way possible.

It is so tempting to see all these references to the crazed, hormonally cycling woman as harmless jokes. But a vast number of studies show that exposure to anything that presents women in these ways develops and maintains gender stereotypes—especially in men. As I'll discuss more in chapter 11, gender stereotypes are widely held and difficult to alter because they are so powerful they shape many aspects of men's and women's lives. This is not only because they are *descriptively* stating what people are like, they are *prescriptively* stating what people "should" be like and "should not" be like.[42]

And when anyone attributes a woman's mood or her anger to PMS rather than the actual situation she's responding to, the opportunity for honest dialog is lost whether in the home, at work, in world affairs, or broadcasted in any media form. Men don't have to do the complicated work of communication and negotiation, and a woman's feelings and thoughts are conveniently invalidated and ignored. This creates a communication chasm that hinders so very much: the development of emotional intimacy across the kitchen table; the influence of half the population across the public stage; the decision-making power in the boardroom; and any chance of having authentic relationships at all. When a man is angry, we assume there must be a good reason that needs addressing. This facilitates a man being able to wield personal and professional power. When a woman's anger is written off as biological and irrational, her chance at wielding similar power is severely diminished.

# PMS Offers a Card to Get Out of Jail, Free

Not only does PMS make all women crazy, it apparently makes us so crazy we can't be held responsible for our behavior. In mid-1800s England, two women were acquitted from murder charges because of irregularities in their menstrual cycles. Almost a century later, two more British women accused of homicide were acquitted with a PMS defense. When a woman in New York City was accused of child abuse in 1982, she initially tried to blame PMS but after emphatic opposition from the district attorney, she dropped it and agreed to plea to a lesser crime.[43] And in 1991, a Virginia woman successfully used her PMS to get charges dropped for driving erratically and kicking the police officer who pulled her over.[44]

A well-liked cartoon shared on Facebook reinforces the idea that women with PMS can't be held responsible. It says: "Feed a cold and starve a fever but give PMS whatever it wants. Trust me... WHATEVER THE HELL IT WANTS."[45] The implication is that if you don't, all hell will break loose, and you are more to blame than the woman.

An extreme example comes from the 2011 California Milk Processor Board's "Everything I Do is Wrong" campaign, which advertised milk to men as a treatment for his woman's PMS. Pictures of harried men holding cartons of milk appeared in magazines with phrases like "I'm sorry I listened to what you said and not what you meant," "I'm sorry for the things I did or didn't do," "I apologize for letting you misinterpret what I was saying," and the clearest message of all, "We can both blame myself."[46] It was a visual and verbal illustration of the idea that when women act crazy before their periods, they must be humored and excused and humiliatingly "managed" in nonsensical ways by men who have to find ways to cope.

The more these messages get out there, the more people accept them. The more people accept them, the easier it becomes to justify placing limits on women. Just as her hormonal rages get dismissed, so do her facts, her opinions, her competency, her decisions, her strength. This has prevented women from gaining access to power and authority at the highest levels in all spheres of life.[47] Indeed, it has prevented some women from even imagining that they belong in male-dominated domains like executive management, a house of representatives, military operations, or coaching a sport.

There are many consequences of perpetuating this myth, and I'll explore them further in chapter 11. For now, I've teased apart the common storylines enough to give you a closer look at what it is like to begin menstruation, come of age, and be a woman. But these storylines are elaborations on a fact that is ubiquitous and natural: women's bodies have a reproductive system. With some solid research about menarche, perhaps the truth of becoming a woman will start to shine through the muck of the myth.

# REAL DATA ON PUBERTY AND MENTAL HEALTH

The average age that menstruating begins, known as "menarche," is twelve and a half for girls in the US and western Europe—although there is a wide range and a lot of influencing factors. Many girls start their periods at the same age their mothers did, but other factors like race and ethnicity have an influence as well: girls of Hispanic and African descent begin to menstruate somewhat earlier than girls with a European background.

Menarche occurs toward the end of the pubertal process—after the development of breasts and pubic hair, and a growth spurt—but in our culture it is erroneously understood as the major mark of its beginning. Generally speaking, "puberty" refers to the physical growth and hormonal changes that culminate in the ability to reproduce. "Adolescence" refers to a much broader time period, which includes the development of reproductive abilities and also the social and psychological processes that happen during the journey from childhood to adulthood.[48]

When girls are prepared for, and educated about, menstruation as a normal, healthy event—especially by their mothers—they reap many benefits. Daughters whose mothers emotionally support them and celebrate their new period as a rite of passage have more positive experiences when menarche occurs, compared to daughters of mothers who ignore it or express negative attitudes.[49] As adults, these young women view their periods more positively, have a better body image, and are more likely to engage in health behaviors like seeing a gynecologist yearly.[50]

Most Americans think of puberty and adolescence as full of hormone-powered emotional volatility. For years psychologists agreed, labeling these years as a time of "storm and stress."[51] But by the new millennium, many studies had contradicted this conclusion. As a whole, psychologists now view puberty and adolescence for both girls and boys as a positive process that most young people traverse without mental-health problems, and without the abundance of conflict that previously characterized it. Although some developmental steps—like desires to have increased control over physical freedom and family decision-making—may bring turbulence, at least 80 percent of adolescents don't show symptoms of emotional distress or behavioral acting out. Yes, the majority of adolescents admit to breaking a rule at least once, but most don't engage in seriously delinquent behavior. The reality is that many more preteens and teens interact comfortably with their parents, siblings, teachers, and friends than don't.[52]

Yet culturally we still assume it's an awful time, full of conflict and emotional issues—because of hormones. Since everyone who goes through puberty has hormonal fluctuations, and we now know that the vast majority of preteens and teens *don't* suffer from emotional and behavioral problems, it makes sense to conclude that changes in hormones—alone—can't be responsible for the emotional and behavioral problems encountered in adolescence.

Scientific evidence supports this. An exhaustive review of the studies on this topic concluded that changes in reproductive hormones alone have a very small effect on adolescent *behavior*. Instead, thorough evidence shows that adolescent behavior is a complex interplay of timing, circumstances, personality, and biology.[53] Hormones are just one small piece of the puzzle, and they have no effect on mental health.

It is true that adolescents experience a wider range of emotions than adults. Their ups are higher and their lows are lower, but not outside the normal range.[54] This may come as a surprise: adolescents even report feeling "very happy" much more commonly than adults.[55]

## REAL REASONS SOME GIRLS STRUGGLE WITH PUBERTY

The number of girls who do have psychological difficulties after menarche makes them a minority, and the most determinant factor is the timing of their first period. There is evidence that girls who start their periods earlier than average are at a higher risk for several emotional and behavioral problems. Emotionally, these girls are more likely to have lower self-esteem, to be embarrassed by their sexually developed bodies, have bad moods, or develop major depression and eating disorders. Behaviorally, early maturing girls are more likely to have older, delinquent friends and engage in antisocial behaviors like vandalism, shoplifting, and fighting. They are also more inclined to drink, smoke, use illegal substances, and participate in sexual activity.[56]

Even so, there are a few caveats worth considering. Early maturing only predicts antisocial behavior when it is affected by previous individual history. Girls who don't have a history of behavior problems *before* menarche are no more likely to have social problems than girls maturing on time.[57] Also, early-maturing girls whose family life is stable and nurturing have no more risk of using illegal drugs than on-time girls. As might be expected, when girls live in a home with conflict, instability, and neglect, maturing early does increase the chance of acting out, as menarche is a developmental transition that happens without a firm foundation to build from. Race influences things also: early-maturing African-American girls are not at any higher risks for emotional problems or early sexual activity, but their risks for behavioral problems like drinking or smoking are at the same increased rate as early-maturing American girls of European or Hispanic descent.[58]

What this research tells us is that there are wide-ranging individual and social factors that determine a girl's emotions and behaviors after menarche. Comparatively speaking, hormones don't have much influence at all.

Most young girls navigate the beginning of menstruation with few, if any, disturbances. But they learn to expect troublesome symptoms, or discount their own lack of symptoms, because they come to believe this myth: the beginning of menstruation marks the beginning of a lifetime of biological and psychological impairment. As a maturing female, they are now officially cyclically incompetent and unreliable. Most people believe the menstrual cycle wreaks havoc on women's emotional stability not because this is what all—or even most—women experience, but because we are inundated with the portrayal of PMSing women as nasty, out-of-control bitches who cannot be held responsible for their actions. This feeds harmful stereotypes that have huge effects. As you've seen in this chapter, all kinds of sources educate us with this message our entire lives. It's no wonder we believe it.

And so the hormone myth begins.

# CHAPTER 2

# Only Flawed Research and Profit Back PMS

The PMS myth persists even though there is a severe lack of scientific evidence to support it. Despite the fact that the last century has produced a voluminous amount of research that resoundingly shows the menstrual phase has no negative impact on women's cognitive functions,[1] the competence of menstruating women continues to be questioned. From the endless number of messages confirming that PMS is a common affliction, we assume there is a mountain of research to support this medical "truth." But as you'll see in this chapter, no strong consensus exists on the definition, the cause, the treatment, or even the existence, of PMS.

## THE LEGEND OF THE PREMENSTRUAL SHE-DEVIL IS BORN

The story of PMS as we know it began in 1931, when, based on a few case studies of individual women he treated, American gynecologist Robert Frank coined the phrase "premenstrual tension" to describe their experiences. He said, "Their personal suffering is intense and manifests itself in many reckless and sometimes reprehensible actions. Not only do they realize their own suffering, but they feel conscience-stricken toward their husbands and families, knowing well that they are unbearable in their attitude and reactions."[2]

The concept was picked up in the 1950s by an English doctor, Katharina Dalton, who built her career around establishing "premenstrual syndrome" as a disorder.[3] An article she wrote with a colleague describing this concept appeared in the prestigious *British Medical Journal* in 1953.[4] She wrote many books and articles purporting that premenstrual women have a higher risk of failing exams, having car accidents, underperforming in the workplace, and developing acute psychiatric illnesses. Since then, psychologists have repeatedly discredited these claims because of the substantial flaws in her studies' methods and the fact that subsequent, methodologically sound research has found that premenstrual women don't perform worse than average—and sometimes do even better. For example, in one study, Dalton reported that 27 percent of teenage girls had a decrease in test performance during the premenstrual phase,[5] but she didn't test this result to make sure it was not due to chance—a basic tenet in the use of statistics. Also, in the publication of this study, Dalton didn't include that, although 27 percent of the girls had a decrease in performance, 56 percent of the girls showed no change and 17 percent had an increase in performance during the premenstrual phase.[6]

The stereotype of women as bad drivers—which is as old as car-driving itself—has been disproved by studies that show premenstrual women have no different, and sometimes fewer, car accidents than women on average and considerably fewer car accidents than men at any time of the month.[7] The higher car-insurance rates men pay tell us, loud and clear, that men have more accidents than women due to their riskier driving patterns.[8]

But bad science and contradictory findings didn't stop Dalton's concept of premenstrual syndrome (PMS) from spreading and getting attention for decades to come. Several of her books became bestsellers, including *Once a Month*, which was published in the late 1970s. She also pioneered the first clinic in England that specifically treated PMS.[9] When Dalton served as the medical expert in a trial in 1981, she argued successfully that a murder defendant wasn't responsible for her actions because her PMS symptoms were severe.[10] This trial generated massive publicity that permeated the United States also.

Articles appearing throughout the 1980s in mainstream news and fitness, health, and women's magazines focused mainly on PMS as an awful problem that women had to manage.[11] Titles included "Coping with Eve's Curse," "The Return of the Raging Hormones," "Once a Month I'm a Woman Possessed," and "Taming the Shrew Inside of You." While we like to think that medical science uses objective methods to answer questions about health and illness, powerful social trends like this contribute to the validation and construction of an illness. During this decade, an idea that prevailed for most of the twentieth century—that mental disorders arose from deep-seated, unresolved conflicts within childhood experiences and unconscious propulsions—gave way to an assumption that all mental illnesses were a product of biological causes. Drugs were being developed that could bring relief to those suffering from schizophrenia, depression, and anxiety, and the definition of PMS as a mental disorder that had a specifically biological cause—hormones—was a part of the shifting winds of psychiatry and psychology at the time.

PMS fit this new biomedical model of mental illness, which gave it traction as a "real" disorder and contributed to its acceptance as a disease by the medical profession. The normal, healthy menstrual cycle became an illness that every woman suffered from.

## WITH SYMPTOMS THIS VAST, EVERYONE COULD HAVE PMS

A mental disorder is a collection of symptoms that are consistently found together and are so severe that it impacts a person's ability to function. The commonly applied definition of PMS is: "Negative emotional, behavioral, and physical symptoms present from the time of ovulation to menstruation." Across studies during fifty years of research, more than 150 different symptoms have been included in definitions of PMS.[12] Here are just a few.

| | |
|---|---|
| acne | hostility |
| anxiety | increased hunger or thirst |
| bloating | irritability |
| breast tenderness | joint pain |
| bursts of energy | low morale |
| change in sex drive | mood swings |
| changes in appetite | more likely to engage in conflicts |
| changes in sleep | muscle pain |
| constipation | nausea |
| crying spells | poor motor coordination |
| decreased interest in activities | skin changes |
| depression | social withdrawal |
| diarrhea | suicidal thoughts |
| difficulty concentrating | sweet or salty cravings |
| fatigue | tension |
| feeling overwhelmed | vertigo |
| headaches | vomiting |

When psychologists come up with a disorder that is defined so vaguely, the label becomes meaningless. Because with a list of symptoms so long and far-reaching, I could have PMS, you could have PMS, my husband could have PMS, even my dog could be diagnosed with PMS.

Now, I want to be clear that I'm not saying that some women don't get some of these symptoms. I know what you're thinking: "Wait a minute! I really do cry at dumb commercials right before my period and my friend always gets headaches." I'm not negating that; the experiences are real. What I'm saying is that getting some of these many symptoms doesn't amount to a mental disorder. Instead, it's a reflection of a normal biological process that is an essential part of being a woman: reproduction.

It's the medical diagnosis that makes a natural reproductive process a disease that I want to draw attention to. In order to be diagnosed with PMS from the 1950s to 1990, some researchers said you had to have five symptoms, some said three. Some said symptoms had to be highly disturbing to you, but others said mild symptoms were equally important. Some said it mattered when in the menstrual cycle you experienced them, but others said they could happen anytime. Because there was no standardization for the definition of PMS, when psychologists tried to report prevalence rates, their estimates ranged from 5 percent of women to 97 percent of women.[13] Which means almost no one, and almost everyone, gets PMS. It doesn't sound very scientific to me.

# FIVE REASONS PMS RESEARCH WAS WRONG

Adhering to the guidelines of the scientific method is critical to producing accurate study results. To say that "a study showed this to be true" is meaningless if the methods of the study were weak. But no one in the media considers that when reporting a sensational finding. And I believe there is no body of research with weaker methods than the research on PMS. From 1964 to 1990, scientific research on PMS had weaknesses in the methods used that overwhelmingly led to inaccurate, misleading, and just-plain-wrong information. Here are the five biggest problems these studies displayed.[14]

## Retrospective Reporting

Women were asked to describe their PMS symptoms *retrospectively*, which means they were asked to describe feelings experienced in the past. Study subjects were asked questions like "In the two weeks before your last period, were you anxious?" Most people are like me: it's really hard to remember what I did two weeks ago, much less to remember how I was feeling at the time. Looking to the past and relying on memory is widely, scientifically known to produce less accurate responses. It even inflates the reporting of symptoms. Due to the cyclical nature of PMS, best methods in research call for *prospective* reporting, which involves tracking symptoms on a daily basis for at least two menstrual cycles in a row.

## No Standardization in PMS Criteria

Various researchers used different criteria in identifying who had PMS. Some questionnaires focused on physical symptoms, some focused on emotional symptoms. There was no consistency in the duration or timing of symptoms necessary to qualify for a diagnosis. In order to conduct reliable research about any condition, scientists must agree on what specific characteristics make up that condition—so they're all talking about the same thing. The studies conducted during this time had no consistent diagnosis criteria.

## Homogeneity of Researchers and Subjects

The great majority of PMS researchers were white academics from Europe, Australia, and the United States. This limited the scope of questions asked because of the prevailing Western cultural belief that the premenstrual period is rife with negative outcomes; the possibility of positive experiences was not even considered, much less explored. In addition, any information gathered about women's premenstrual experiences was limited by the fact that the subjects being studied were almost exclusively white, European-American, middle-class women. This makes it impossible to apply study findings to all women—but that was exactly what happened.

## Problems with Timing

Studies interviewed women at different times of the month and for one menstrual cycle only. But it's universally understood that PMS involves recurring symptoms during the luteal phase of the menstrual cycle, from ovulation to menstruation. Despite this, PMS studies assessed women's symptoms at a variety of phases in their cycle—making it impossible to attribute symptoms to any particular phase of the month. Furthermore, most studies interviewed women for one menstrual cycle only, when the best way to determine if a cyclical syndrome exists is to measure symptoms for several consecutive cycles to confirm a pattern.

## Not Using Control Groups

Including a control group is one of the most critical parts of carrying out a valid study. A control group includes participants who ideally experience everything the same as the experimental group, except the variable being tested. But across the board, PMS research was done on women who believed they had PMS. Having a control group of women who *don't* identify as having PMS would provide a baseline of outcome variables to compare to women who *do* identify as having PMS, so that experiences could be more accurately assessed as they do or don't relate to symptoms. Control groups also help eliminate the influence that naturally occurring differences among people—like personal history, pain sensitivity, personality, or life events—can have on how they report symptoms. And it also mitigates the influence of outside variables, like exposure to media messages and popular culture.[15] By not using control groups, researchers effectively removed any context with which to interpret the study findings. For example, if the results of a study show that women with PMS have elevated depressive symptoms, the question is: elevated compared to whom? To be able to say that any symptoms were elevated because of PMS, researchers need to be able to illustrate that women who are similar in every way, except having PMS, have lower depressive symptoms. And the most effective way to do that is to include a control group.

The idea that women's emotions are dictated by their reproductive organs is ancient and, once PMS was established in the medical profession as a diagnosable illness, scientific researchers dropped the methods that preserve the objectivity of unbiased data. Both medical and psychological researchers applied the scientific method to PMS studies in haphazard ways, resulting in a body of research more flawed than almost any other subject.

Their findings have had incredible power over the psychological and physical health treatment of women. Katharina Dalton was a major proponent of progesterone therapy as a treatment for PMS and provided it to her patients for many years. The successes she reported with individual patients were covered by the popular media—50 percent of the PMS articles I mentioned earlier in this chapter discussed progesterone as a treatment.[16] But later clinical trials of large groups of women—a much more reliable method than individual cases—didn't produce any convincing evidence of progesterone's effectiveness. Progesterone comes with many potential side effects that range from nausea and depression to increased risk of cancer and heart disease. As I'll discuss more in chapter 10, women receiving this treatment put their health at risk.

By the mid-1990s and early 2000s, significant methodological improvements were made in this field of research, with some fascinating results. By 1994, after a huge influx of female researchers entered the field of psychology, a groundbreaking study was conducted that showed the power of simply allowing for the possibility of a positive aspect of menstruation. Fifty female college students completed a questionnaire that asked them to rate how often they experience joyful symptoms around menstruation, such as feelings of increased sexual desire, excitement, and bursts of energy. Then they completed another questionnaire about their attitudes on menstruation. The subjects who were simply exposed to the idea that some women might experience positive changes reported more positive attitudes about menstruation compared to those who weren't given that idea. After completing the "menstrual joy questionnaire," 30 percent of the women said that it had made them think about menstruation in a different way.[17]

The fact that PMS is nearly unheard of outside of Western nations[18] shows how strongly this cultural bias influenced supposedly scientific research. When finally studied, Chinese women reported no premenstrual emotional upset along with the physical symptoms of cycling they did report like fatigue, water retention, pain, and increased sensitivity to cold.[19] When researchers studied women in India, they reported few to no premenstrual difficulties[20] and viewed menstruation as generally positive.[21]

## RESEARCH METHODS IMPROVED, SO WHO HAS PMS NOW?

While as a culture we remain trapped in a myth established and supported by bad science, the science itself has moved on. In 1994, the fourth edition of the *Diagnostic and Statistical Manual of Mental Disorders* (DSM-4) was published. As the manual psychologists must use to diagnose mental health illnesses, the new edition made waves by transforming the PMS diagnosis into "premenstrual dysphoric disorder" (PMDD). At last, a more clear-cut definition of this experience emerged with specific symptoms and distinct conditions required for a diagnosis. The DSM-4 accomplished this by applying five levels of criteria for diagnosis.

First, the new diagnosis guidelines narrowed the symptoms. A woman has to suffer at least one of these four: feeling noticeably depressed, anxious, moody, or irritable. She also has to experience at least four more symptoms which might be one of those above, or from a list of seven types of symptoms like feeling lethargic, finding concentration difficult, having trouble sleeping, or experiencing some of the common physical complaints like bloating or breast tenderness. This change alone brought great progress in putting an end to diagnosing anyone and everyone who has a female reproductive system with a mental disorder. If you don't have five of the possible eleven symptoms, you don't have PMDD.

Second, the required timing of the symptoms became very specific. To receive a diagnosis of PMDD, a woman has to experience symptoms during the week before menstruation starts and she has to get better by the time menstruation ends. This helps doctors considering this diagnosis be sure they apply it to women who feel these symptoms exclusively in the premenstrual period.

Third, the new guidelines cut back on the number of women who were labeled with a disorder just because they recalled that one month in the past they felt cranky or sad before they got their period. That's not mental illness, that's a normal fluctuation of mood. To be diagnosed with PMDD, women must have cyclical symptoms recur for at least three menstrual cycles in a row, which has to be confirmed by daily documentation of symptoms throughout the month.

Fourth, a woman not only has to experience the symptoms, they have to disturb her ability to function socially or professionally. This is a classic defining element of any mental disorder, and it is vital to separate women who are simply having a bad day from those whose symptoms are overwhelming their ability to carry on in life.

Finally, the new criteria eliminated the possibility that the symptoms observed were due to an already-existing disorder. Illnesses like major depression or bipolar disorder can have some similarities to PMDD, but are not necessarily cyclical and require different treatment. This is an important caveat to the diagnosis because it impacts appropriate client care.

Neither my husband nor my dog can be diagnosed with PMDD. Psychologists evaluating clients and researchers exploring treatments are now talking about the same thing, which makes research more reliable and consistent. Using this more stringent criteria, studies are overwhelmingly showing that, on average, *between 3 to 8 percent of women* suffer from PMDD.[22] Not all women, not most women, not a majority of women, not even a lot of women—just 3 to 8 percent. For everyone else, many other variables like stressful events, happy occasions, even the day of the week are more powerful predictors of mood than hormone level or phase of the menstrual cycle.[23]

This is information the scientific community has had since the late 1980s and early 1990s. Many psychologists have published articles documenting the flawed PMS research and low prevalence rate of PMDD, in the process protesting PMS as a diagnostic label and establishing PMDD as a helpful diagnosis for women who truly are debilitated and affected in life-altering ways by their monthly cycle.[24] The question we have to ask is no longer why all women have PMS, but rather why this information about PMDD hasn't trickled into public conversation in the decades that have passed since it began emerging. Well, here's where the story begins to thicken. The rest of this chapter and the entire chapter that follows explore the question: Why does the PMS myth persist despite the evidence?

## THE EFFECTS OF BEING DIAGNOSED WITH A MENTAL ILLNESS

As I enter this discussion, it's important for you to keep in mind what happens when someone is given a diagnosis. On the positive side, the designation of a collection of symptoms as an official disorder validates what people are experiencing as "real," and, particularly in the Internet age, helps them to find a community that shares these symptoms so they can receive practical advice and empathy. The relief of finding out they're not suffering alone can be very powerful, which is true for many women who suffer the debilitating symptoms of PMDD. By establishing a clear diagnosis, the debilitating experiences that some women have are acknowledged and validated; they don't have to question themselves or worry whether "it's all in my head." The establishment of the PMDD diagnosis also increases the reliability of research on it, makes its causes more accurately discernable, and contributes to the development of effective treatments.

Now the downside: we don't have very positive images of people with mental disorders, so those who are diagnosed can be stigmatized and isolated. In our individualistic, pull-yourself-up-by-the-bootstraps society, common perceptions may interpret people as weak or just not trying hard enough. People with mental illnesses are commonly portrayed in the media as disheveled, incompetent, and criminal. Depending on the condition, an insurance company can deny or limit certain kinds of coverage, like disability or life insurance, if a psychiatric diagnosis from the DSM is in medical records. Divorce courts can even deny custody of children on the same basis.

A diagnosis makes it much more likely that the patient will be prescribed medication, since that form of treatment has become the most common type of psychological aid. These drugs are effective to varying degrees and most psychological drugs come with side effects, ranging from the mildly annoying to the debilitating.[25] A common treatment prescribed for PMDD is a class of antidepressants called SSRIs that include Prozac and Celexa. For these drugs, mild side effects like nausea and sleeplessness generally dissipate over time, but they also commonly cause a decrease in libido and the ability to have an orgasm—something women might miss a lot. Hormone therapy, in the form of oral contraceptives or estrogen alone, is also commonly prescribed for PMDD, although there is little consistent evidence for its effectiveness.[26] Hormone therapy, as I discuss in depth in chapter 10, is known to raise the risk for cancer, heart disease, and other circulatory disorders.

## DIAGNOSING MENTAL DISORDERS IN WOMEN

You might think psychologists base the diagnosis of a mental disorder on scientific evidence, but science makes up only a small part of the story. For most of the twentieth century, doctors who were predominantly white and male established the existence of a disorder by reflecting on what they observed in patients and then conferring with other psychologists to come to a consensus. Their consensus created our definitions of mental health and mental disease.

This consensual approach guided the first two editions of the DSM. Its authority in diagnosing mental disorders is similar to that of the *Physician's Desk Reference* for medical disorders. Published and owned by the American Psychiatric Association, the DSM creates clear-cut categories that designate behaviors as ranging from the merely eccentric to reflecting a mental illness, and can have a tremendous impact on many aspects of a person's life, which include validating personal experience and also imposing the crippling stigmas I described in the last section.[27] Scholars have deeply criticized the common practice of measuring women's mental health against the long-held standard of a healthy human: the white, heterosexual male. Before the 1970s, when more women became psychologists and psychiatrists, the "experts" routinely labeled women's behavior as disordered or deficient when compared to a male standard.[28]

After World War II, Freudian theories of mental health viewed women as less mentally healthy because of their inevitable penis envy and considered a woman to be mentally disturbed if she rejected the typically feminine roles of wife and mother. These ideas were widely accepted, to the degree that their misogyny was treated as fact. Throughout the 1950s, 60s, and 70s, if a woman sought help with depression because of dissatisfaction with the domestic life of child-rearing and homemaking, she was likely to be prescribed a tranquilizer like Valium, or told to "go buy a new hat."[29]

One excellent analysis of the popular media of the 1950s describes how the development and ensuing popularity of a tranquilizer called Miltown reflected the perception that fulfilling the feminine role was essential to conceptions of women's mental health. The examination of advertisements for, and articles about, Miltown in magazines like *Newsweek, Ladies' Home Journal,* and *Science Digest* from 1955 to 1969 found that it was popular to discuss women's frustrations with the hyper-feminine ideal of the time and the fact that many women wanted to remain in the jobs they had undertaken during World War II. But within these ads and articles, women's unhappinesses and anxieties were not the major concerns being addressed—rather, they spoke to the isolation and dissatisfaction that men felt, making these the true problems that needed fixing. Readers were told that tranquilizers could make frigid women respond to their husbands and could even return a psychotic woman to her household responsibilities—as if mopping the floor indicated good mental health, even if she did hear voices while doing it. Anxious, unresponsive women who refused to do housework were simply unacceptable to society.[30]

This thinking was the foundation for the popularity of PMS because this disorder also conveyed that, if a woman is angry or unsatisfied and therefore making her man miserable, her experience must be called a disease and treated. PMS was—and continues to be—a way to turn a woman's anger and frustration into a mental illness.

With her 1972 book *Women and Madness*, psychologist Phyllis Chesler challenged the gendered way that mental illness had been defined. She revealed that what had been labeled as symptoms of mental illness in women would be more accurately characterized as "violations of feminine norms of behavior." In her interviews with women in psychiatric institutions, some women reported that they had been institutionalized by their families because they were too "troublesome" or had a "fighting spirit."[31] Chesler's book was a harbinger of the shift from the common male-centered view of women to a more complex understanding of women's lives.[32] Spurred by the women's movement, the influx of women into the field of psychology in this decade brought new perspectives on women's mental health. Female psychologists studied topics that had been previously ignored such as domestic violence, women's achievement needs, and sexual harassment.[33] The feminist movement of the 1970s, and all that was learned because of it, demanded that we stop pretending that a new hat was all a woman needed to be happy.

## THE HEATED DISCUSSION BEHIND DSM REVISIONS

The first edition of the DSM that was published in 1952 described each recognized disorder and its identifying symptoms based primarily on practitioner expertise, since applying the scientific method to mental health was not the norm. By the publication of the DSM-3 in 1980 and the DSM-3-R in 1987, the philosophical basis behind the definition of mental disorders had shifted from professional expertise to empirical research with a biomedical emphasis.[34] However, changes in the DSM don't always follow this new philosophy.

The process of assessing the inclusion of PMS and PMDD within the DSM has always been politically charged.[35] PMS did not appear as a disorder in the first three editions and when revisions were prepared for the DSM-3-R, a committee was created to establish whether or not adding it to the list of disorders was merited by empirical research and was clinically useful. When it became clear that the committee intended to recommend that PMS should be listed as a disorder, it came under considerable criticism.

As I previously discussed, the effect of labeling something a disorder in the DSM can alter many lives, as we saw vividly with homosexuality. For most of the twentieth century, homosexuality was seen as representing deviant feelings and behavior. Because the first two editions of the DSM listed it as an official mental disorder, many men and women were subjected to hospitalization and treatments that ranged from psychoanalysis and aversion therapy to castration and clitoridectomies—often without consent.[36] The American Psychiatric Association removed the "homosexual" category from the DSM-3-R not because of any change in empirical research, but because of the political pressure brought by gay-rights activists and the evolving cultural acceptance of homosexuality as a naturally occurring sexual orientation.

When it came to the PMS debate, many groups of mental health professionals, including the American Psychological Association, the American Psychiatric Association Committee on Women, and the National Association of Social Workers, protested against its inclusion for three reasons: there was little research to support its inclusion; the new category would erroneously label women as mentally ill; and it would effectively stigmatize women and reinforce old stereotypes of women as hormonal and irrational.[37] Few saw an advantage to implying scientific validation for the image of women as raging, hormonal lunatics.

After much debate within the committee and pressure from feminist groups like NOW, the committee proposed a much more specific and debilitating version of PMS that they called "late luteal premenstrual dysphoric disorder" (LLPDD), with "late luteal" referring to the specific time after ovulation but before menstruation begins, and "dysphoria" meaning a feeling of unease or depression. This disorder was added to the appendix of the DSM-3-R in a list of disorders in need of further study. By the publication of the DSM-4 in 1994, LLPDD was renamed PMDD and it appeared in the main text, which reflected a body of research that had developed under more stringent guidelines.[38]

The establishment of an official mental illness is messy business and is the product of professional, scientific, and social influences. The publication of the DSM and its subsequent revisions simultaneously brings positive and negative consequences to those it labels mentally ill. When researchers realize which of their assumptions are based on flawed science, there is always the possibility for improved clarity and understanding like we have seen with the more rigorous and specific reconceptualization of PMS as PMDD. It has made research on prevalence and treatment much more valid and reliable. It bears repeating that, now that we are using a more clear-cut definition, the prevalence of this disorder has plummeted from previous estimates of up to 97 percent of menstruating women to only 3 to 8 percent. But despite the convincing evidence that should have brought the hormone myth's demise, PMS storylines persist. We need to look farther afield to find out why.

## THE PROFIT MOTIVE

With the majority of childbearing-aged women believing they suffer from a monthly illness, a gigantic client base exists that can be endlessly tapped. PMS treatment is a thriving, profitable industry—on many fronts. Simply legitimizing PMS as a disorder opened the door for money to be made, starting with the American Psychiatric Association, which publishes the DSM. Critics of the DSM argue that disorders like PMDD are added with more of a motive for profit than for enhancing mental health. When the authors add or change disorders, revised editions—there have been seven—necessitate repeated purchases by practitioners and researchers[39] and bring in about $5 million per year.[40] So the new editions need to appeal to as broad a market as possible, and many argue that they draw on popular discourse far too much.

Adding disorders is also an economic boon to mental health practitioners because it creates more "sick" people in need of treatment.[41] Recognized disorders are reimbursed by health insurance companies, ensuring practitioners will get paid. In 2013, the DSM-5 added "caffeine withdrawal" as a new disorder.[42] Yes, cutting off a coffee habit is hard, but suddenly it's a mental disorder? This practice of labeling any annoying or difficult aspect of life as pathological is becoming more common, with few advantages for the patient. It creates an unrealistically perfect version of health and encourages people to focus on and evaluate every unpleasant sensation. Rather than understanding minor difficulties as commonplace and generally meaningless, we now obsess and turn our energy and focus from the concerns and activities of the outside world to the minor complaints of our inner world.

Pharmaceutical companies benefit from a diagnosis the most. When the DSM legitimizes disorders, pharmaceutical companies can develop and sell new drugs to treat them. Also, existing drugs can be repurposed to expand on an already-established clientele. When the DSM-5 added "restless leg syndrome" as a disorder, sales of the drug Mirapex increased. Previously, doctors had prescribed it to alleviate symptoms of Parkinson's disease, but suddenly it had a whole new market because of a newly validated disorder.[43] The pharmaceutical industry is enormously profitable; prescription drug sales brought in $326 billion in 2014 alone.[44]

It won't surprise anyone who watches television or reads magazines that pharmaceutical companies spend twice as much on advertising as they do on the research and development of new treatments.[45] Ads for prescription drugs, directed at consumers—not doctors—have become an integral part of their sales strategy. Studies show that doctors are substantially more likely to prescribe something when a patient asks for it by name, particularly when it comes to antidepressants.[46] That is how this industry maintains one of the highest profit margins of all American industries.

## ANYTHING DIAGNOSABLE NEEDS MEDS, WHETHER HELPFUL OR NOT

Here's what happened when the DSM-4 gave PMDD a diagnosis code. The pharmaceutical company Eli Lilly had a long, profitable run with the antidepressant that was marketed as Prozac and known generically as fluoxetine. At its height, Prozac was bringing in almost $3 billion in annual sales.[47] But in 1999, their patent on fluoxetine was about to run out and, if it did, other pharmaceutical companies would be able to sell generic versions and Eli Lilly would lose the monopoly it had with Prozac. To extend their exclusive hold on the market, Eli Lilly applied to the FDA to approve fluoxetine as a treatment for PMDD so they could market it anew as Sarafem.

In the application, they presented the FDA with a review paper— which examines all of the studies done on a particular question in a recent time period to reach a broad conclusion—that supported treating PMDD with fluoxetine.[48] But the majority of the studies the authors cited to support their conclusion came from the flawed, inconsistent research on PMS that was conducted before the DSM established the more stringent criteria for PMDD. Also, Eli Lilly funded the writing of the paper—a huge reason to suspect its impartiality. Despite this, the FDA approved their application that same year.[49] This kept annual sales above $2 billion for three more years, a total windfall for the pharmaceutical company.

Yet, the FDA's approval may have actually hurt women. Leading psychologists of women's reproductive health documented three ways this happened.[50]

## Rebranding to Mislead

Eli Lilly misled women by renaming Prozac in order to sidestep women's concerns about taking the antidepressant at a time when concerns over the drug—and antidepressants in general—were being loudly expressed. Without the word Prozac in sight, the rebranded Sarafem even comes in a girly pink and purple box.

## Increasing Risk for Known Side Effects

Although the FDA ruled that Prozac was safe to use for PMDD patients, it has many commonly experienced side effects, including nausea, headaches, anxiety, insomnia, and sexual dysfunction. While risking these side effects may be justifiable when treating severe depression, when women take on the chance of having them because they've been encouraged to confuse mild premenstrual symptoms with full-blown PMDD, the risks become excessive.[51]

## Convincing All Women to See Themselves as Mentally Ill

The extensive Sarafem marketing campaign that hit television, the Internet, and women's magazines confused the concept of PMS with the portrayal of PMDD in order to convince women they are mentally ill. Sarafem ads effectively portray *physical* premenstrual symptoms as indicative of mental illness, which takes a small minority of women that studies show have PMDD and make it appear that the vast majority need mental health treatment.

When other pharmaceutical companies gained permission to sell treatments for PMDD, their advertising campaigns reasserted this message over and over again. The ads for Paxil run by the company GlaxoSmithKline said, "I always thought it was just PMS. Now I know otherwise. Grouchy? Emotional? Irritable? It may be PMDD."[52]

## HORMONE THERAPY PROFITS FROM MYTH, NOT SCIENCE

Another sizable source of revenue for pharmaceutical companies is the sale of reproductive hormones to alleviate the confused blend of PMS and PMDD symptoms. These are the active ingredients in oral contraceptives, better known as birth-control pills, because they are prescribed to prevent pregnancy. But they have overwhelming appeal to mitigate symptoms of PMS and PMDD, including mood stabilization. Hormone therapy is incredibly popular, even though studies repeatedly find that low levels of progesterone don't alleviate symptoms. In 2009, the *Harvard Review of Psychiatry* published a review of studies that examined the effectiveness of progesterone alone, and also of medications that combine both estrogen and progesterone, to treat PMS and PMDD. And it concluded that there is little evidence of effectiveness.[53] Only two studies have compared women treated with oral contraceptives to a control group of women treated with placebos and both studies showed that they had no effect on relieving PMDD symptoms.[54] Hormone therapy comes with serious risks. It can lead to heart disease and breast cancer, something I'll discuss more in chapter 10.

According to FDA regulations, for a drug to be deemed effective, a large portion of the target population should experience improvement of symptoms.[55] If PMS were actually a distinct disorder with a distinct cause, large numbers of women should benefit from the treatments developed. Clearly, PMDD treatments don't meet that standard. But having women convinced they are sick and that a simple pill, taken once a day, will make them better creates an enormous market that brings billion-dollar profits.

# RIDING THE MYTH WITH
# OVER-THE-COUNTER TREATMENTS

Drugs bought over the counter, like Midol, promise to treat PMS symptoms like tension and irritability—even though they only contain a pain reliever, a diuretic, and caffeine.[56] While we can all agree that caffeine has magical powers, few would experience it as *reducing* tension since it has been widely shown to heighten anxiety. Some women say that these kinds of over-the-counter drugs bring them relief, and it's likely to be the case because the ingredients do ease pain. Being uncomfortable or in pain can put a damper on anyone's mood, so easing that pain will undoubtedly make a woman feel better.

Since 2002, Teen Midol has been advertised to teenage girls through e-mail and the Internet to convince them early that everyone gets PMS and that it will make you a monster for the rest of your life. But wait! There's something you can do about it: take Midol and you will be a reasonable human being again.[57] The hope is that these girls will do this every month for a lifetime—and there's nothing so coveted as a lifelong customer. In 2012, this approach took in $48 million in sales revenue.[58]

Another business that profits tremendously from the myth of widespread PMS is the Wild West industry of dietary supplements. With retail sales of $28 billion in 2014, selling alternative medications to consumers is big business.[59] Common vitamins and minerals recommended for PMS treatment include vitamin $B_6$, calcium, magnesium, and manganese—with little evidence that they provide relief or are safe for women to take. Herbal products such as evening primrose oil, chasteberry, and St. John's Wort are also sold to treat PMS symptoms, although their effectiveness is questionable and their safety has not been well established.[60]

The effectiveness of any treatment of PMS has been difficult to determine because of the vague way PMS has been defined. Nevertheless, the unregulated industry of dietary supplements has advertised and sold many PMS treatments to women. Studies comparing women taking evening primrose oil with control groups of women taking placebos have found inconsistent effectiveness results. And some have shown no added benefit to taking evening primrose oil over a placebo in relieving PMDD symptoms.[61] The use of chasteberry is not safe during pregnancy and therefore shouldn't be used if a woman may become pregnant.[62] And these supplements don't come cheap. Combination supplements claiming to treat PMS that contain vitamins, minerals, and herbs can cost between twenty-five and eighty dollars per bottle.[63]

# CLINICS AND SEMINARS AND WORKSHOPS, OH MY!

Who else has made money on PMS and PMDD? Medical practitioners. A quick Google search on PMS treatment brings up a cornucopia of clinics, seminars, and workshops. The fact that researchers have never been able to establish the cause of PMS or PMDD is reflected in the fact that so many different kinds of medical practitioners offer treatment. Clinics are run by gynecologists, endocrinologists, psychologists, chiropractors, nurse practitioners, and nutritionists.[64]

Although the websites for these clinics gain authority from the staffs' medical degrees, the information provided about PMS and PMDD is not scientific. The websites describe PMS as a known disorder that includes up to 150 different symptoms and that affects 90 to 95 percent of women[65]—stats I hope I've shown you are all false. Some websites suggest PMS plays a role in marital strife and child abuse.[66] Now the raging hormonal beast not only makes her husband miserable, but beats her children too? These are not facts by any means; they are sensational exaggerations. They epitomize the manipulative disinformation used to convince women that they are dangerous and sick, and that "science" can cure them if they just get help from medical professionals and buy unproven treatments. Some clinics even offer high-interest-rate payment plans for treatment—a highly profitable practice.[67] The need to finance medical treatment is often associated with elective treatments not deemed medically necessary and therefore not covered by insurance.[68]

But the money doesn't explain it all. Who else benefits from the myth of the raging hormonal woman? The next chapter explores how those in power have trotted out the concept of PMS whenever women have tried to overstep the boundaries implied by their gender. And, while an unsettling idea, I'll discuss how women gain social benefits from attributing anger or irritability to their PMS.

# CHAPTER 3

# Keeping Women Down, Each and Every Month

In 1976, the physician Edgar Berman famously said, "Take a woman surgeon. If she had premenstrual tension—and people with this frequently end up in a psychiatrist's office—I wouldn't want her operating on me."[1] This statement illustrates how the assumption that menstrual cycles make women crazy has been a powerful tool for limiting their opportunities and, by default, maintaining the greater status of men. The basis of the whole discussion is a thought that goes even further back than Aristotle, but which he clearly expressed: that women are inferior to men.

The myth of widespread PMS perpetuates this idea in our current worldview by setting up a duality between male and female qualities. At heart, it has us believe that males are essentially reason-based in their behavior—which brings consistency and competence. Whereas women are emotion-based in their behavior, and therefore unpredictable and unreliable.[2]

In so very many contexts and situations, the myth makes it possible to put down, minimize, and invalidate any woman. Even thinking that a woman who is angry, aggressive, or assertive might be on her period stamps what she has said with a big, red-inked message: "unreliable." It reinforces the biases we all have, which look out for any evidence that a woman is less accurate and stable than men. The menstruation accusation, whether stated or not, is a disarming and disempowering tool that these days is wielded by men and women alike.

The tremendous staying power of the PMS myth—despite no evidence to support its reality—is an ongoing, cultural confirmation that women are "cunning," "manipulative," "hysterical," and "irrational."[3]

This chapter looks at ways this has been used to limit women in family life, at work, and within themselves.

## THE DOCILE IDEAL

Labeling menstruation as a disease accomplishes two things: it rejects women's rebelliousness and keeps women in their place.[4] During the era of bad science I described in the last chapter, commonly cited symptoms in the premenstrual stage included the inability, or unwillingness, to care for others and carry out domestic tasks like cooking and cleaning.[5] Culturally, we know that being a good woman involves always putting the needs of others first—any Mother's Day card can tell you that with sentiments like "Mom, you've always been there." Central to a woman's ability to achieve this ideal of perpetual emotional availability is to maintain emotional self-control. A good woman controls and subverts her own needs. Women are expected to keep it together and stay buttoned-up for the sake of everyone else.

Ideal female qualities of submissiveness and sacrifice were reinforced with the advent of the industrial revolution. In the early nineteenth century, the average American family's daily life changed from agricultural tasks—in which men and women worked side by side to ensure the family's survival, both active and productive—to industrial capitalist tasks. When men left the home to earn a wage in the savage, cold, cruel marketplace, women were no longer needed to grind the wheat to make the bread that fed the family, nor to make the clothes on their backs. These could all be provided by the marketplace. Women, particularly white and middle- or upper-class women, had to find a new purpose.[6]

The answer to the "woman question" was something that has been called the "cult of true womanhood" or the "cult of domesticity." If this new economy required a man to be rational, self-focused, and ambitious, a woman should be the opposite. The four major attributes of true womanhood were piety, purity, submissiveness, and domesticity.[7] While men were the doers and actors in society, women were expected to be passive and submissive with the purpose of creating a warm, conflict-free oasis to which her husband could retreat. This standard of womanhood was relayed through magazines and the religious writings of the time. One book advised brides to embrace this submission as the will of God: "Oh, young and lovely bride, watch well the first moments when your will conflicts with his to whom God and society have given the control. Reverence his wishes even when you do not his opinions."[8] *Godey's Lady's Book*, one of the most popular women's magazines of the 1850s, confirmed the grim reality of the ideal that women had to reach for with messages like "[t]o suffer and be silent under suffering seems the great command she has to obey."[9]

The oppression women felt under this ideal of submission and inactivity was searingly described in Charlotte Perkins Gilman's short story "The Yellow Wallpaper," published in 1892. It is a semiautobiographical account of Gilman's struggle: before she got married, she had been a financially independent writer and was devoted to public service. She hesitated to enter into marriage for fear it would limit her ability to be an active person in society. Her fears were realized when she plunged into depression after the birth of her first child and was prescribed the infamous "rest cure." This popular treatment for a variety of women's mental illnesses involved lying in bed for most, if not all, hours of the day, secluded, with a total lack of activity—especially intellectual activity. Gilman wrote that three months of this "cure" nearly drove her insane; she only found relief when she "cast the noted specialist's advice to the winds and went to work again."[10]

## KEEPING WOMEN WORKERS EXPENDABLE

From the time PMS was introduced in 1931, it was used to support the belief that a woman's ability to do good work was compromised at key moments in American history: whenever women were perceived to be taking men's jobs.[11] Robert Frank published his original paper on premenstrual tension in these conditions, after the majority of men had been away fighting World War I and the number of working women had increased. When the men returned, the harsh economic conditions of the Great Depression ensued, and government and corporate policies were formed to compel women to leave the workforce so men could take those jobs.

Many social analysts have pointed to the coinciding timing between the emergence of studies showing the debilitating effects of the menstrual cycle on work productivity and the belief that women's participation in the labor force was an obstacle to men's full employment.[12] So it begins to make sense that, when men left to fight in World War II and labor needs were high to sustain the war effort, many studies came out that found menstruation had *no* ill effect on women's productivity. A review of the studies from that era found that menstruation was not associated with job performance, production, or absenteeism, and that menstruation itself caused no incapacity.[13] But when men returned from the battlefield, social pressure rose for women to make way for them—establishing a theme of the expendability of women in the workforce. This was when Katharina Dalton's research spread popularly, with her faulty claims that PMS reduced women's cognitive abilities, and made them clumsy and accident-prone.[14]

In the early part of the twentieth century, the increase in employ-ment opportunities for women was the result of the military's need for the men who would normally have filled these jobs. But the story of the great influx of women entering the working world in the latter part of the same century is much, much different; in the 1970s, it was caused by a revolu-tionary social movement to expand traditional gender roles.[15] As this movement led to the percentage of working women shooting from 37 percent in 1960 to 52 percent in 1980,[16] those who were committed to keeping women in traditional, domestic roles bolstered their arguments by perpetuating the myth of rampant PMS. Katharina Dalton's writings during this time emphasize women's responsibility to get treatment and return to their rightful role in the family and home, "otherwise they will get what they deserve from their husbands."[17]

This time, however, women didn't leave the workforce. They were there to stay, and continued to increase their numbers in both business and higher education. So it shouldn't be a surprise that in the late 1970s and early 1980s, there was an eruption of research and media that focused on PMS. Once again, it was described as a common affliction that—among other effects that burdened everyone—lowered women's perfor-mance at school and work.[18]

In chapter 3, I went deep into the unbelievably flawed and unreliable PMS studies of this era. Drawing on that, and on historical patterns, we can see a cultural effort at play. The regularity of this "scientific" response to women's advancements into the realms of men reveals the social agenda behind it: to protect male domination over the working world and to keep women docile and in the home.[19]

# "WOMEN ARE RUINING THEIR OWN LIVES"

The conservative shift of the Reagan Era stoked these ideas and supported labeling PMS as an illness all women have. It resulted in a concerted political and cultural backlash against feminists and women's advancement in general. Led by Christian fundamentalist ministers like Jerry Falwell, the founder of the Moral Majority, this ideology was popularized: a man should be the head of the family, a wife should be submissive to her husband, and a woman's most important role is to be a mother. Falwell claimed that feminists, with their work toward gender equality and women's participation in the workforce, had ruined family life in a "satanic attack on the home."

This concept that feminism had ruined the lives of women, men, and children was reinforced by unfounded media stories about an "infertility epidemic" and "toxic daycare." Television shows portrayed career women as sabotaging their own happiness. In *thirtysomething*, the character named Hope was a stay-at-home mom presented in the most positive light: thoughtful, loving, and completely satisfied to be home caring for her husband and child. The other female characters, not as domestically oriented as Hope, were not given such an angelic aura. Melissa was a struggling and single photographer who was likeable, but pathetic, neurotic, miserable, and pining for the domestic bliss of Hope and her husband. Ellyn was a highly successful public official, but was portrayed as harsh and selfish for devoting herself to her career. She was distinctly not maternal and not that interested in romantic relationships. She paid a heavy price for her devotion to her job; the writers gave her a bleeding ulcer that showed how her ambition destroyed her health. And the most unlikeable personality was reserved for the acerbic Susannah, a single feminist and social activist who is mean, heartless, and humorless. Her independence is mocked by the other characters and she has no redeeming qualities.

The writers' messages were clear: good women want to be maternal and domestic, bad women are ambitious and career-oriented, and these bad women are ruining their own lives.[20] Abundant media from this era similarly portray working women as harried, mean, selfish, and unfulfilled. It gave us negative images to draw on that reinforced a surrender to our maternal bodies, our giving natures, and our limitations as women. In many ways, PMS has been made out as something we are doomed to suffer as a reminder that we don't belong in the world of men because our biologically-based mothering ability, and our professional excellence, are mutually exclusive.

## THE DAY-TO-DAY REALITY OF MOTHERING

Motherhood brings with it another standard of womanhood many women find unreachable: the happy, satisfied, uncomplaining mother. Feminists call this ideal "the motherhood mystique," and define it as "The popular beliefs that motherhood is natural, easy, and always enjoyable, and that optimal child development requires a mother's full-time dedication."[21]

Women know the tremendous effort childcare requires. Especially when caring for very young children, it can be physically draining, thankless work. Raising children is a complex endeavor, with highs and lows that often feel chaotic and messy, and that requires split-second responses that keep caregivers forever on their toes. Even with the bright moments and wisps of appreciation, a day with the children can be exhausting.

But it is forbidden to voice negative feelings about mothering responsibilities. A good mother is defined by her willingness to sacrifice for her loved ones, so any mother who complains, yells, or talks about needing to escape her duties for just a day can be branded a "bad mother." This is probably the worst thing you can call a woman. While she loves her children dearly, they challenge her left and right, in all ways. So when a woman can't keep up the "good mother" standard, she blames her behavior on PMS, which allows her to assure others that this state is temporary—and not her real self.[22]

## THE FULL PLATE OF TODAY'S WOMAN

In this modern age, when 58.6 percent of the 123 million American women ages 16 years and over were labor force participants—working or looking for work[23]—expectations of women are high and multitudinous. To many, the ideal woman is: educated and successful in her career; an attractive, supportive partner to her spouse; a doting, generous mother; a housekeeper; a diplomat in family relations; and a de facto caregiver to the sick and the old. That is one full plate.

The good news is that, overall, women with multiple roles and responsibilities have increased physical and psychological well-being. But research shows that when those roles become overwhelming and women feel unsupported, they suffer from stress and strain.[24] Women sometimes negotiate this strain by using PMS as an acceptable reason for withdrawing from their usually required responsibilities, especially domestic chores.[25] Studies show that PMS allows them to renegotiate the many roles they inhabit.[26]

On the face of it, asking a husband to take on household chores might seem to some as a rebellious, feminist act. But with close to 60 percent of women at work and contributing to the family income, traditional roles are shifting: in 2014, on an average day, 20 percent of men reported doing housework—such as cleaning or doing laundry—compared with 49 percent of women. Forty-three percent of men did food preparation or cleanup activities versus 69 percent of women.[27] So while men are sharing more of the housework, the bulk of it still falls to women. This is why framing a request for help with PMS symptoms—basically asking for temporary relief from being overburdened in the name of PMS—changes the perceived nature of the request. Instead of risking coming across as demanding, overbearing, complaining, or a nag, women can instead be victims of their hormones who are reaching out for help.

## THE NEED TO VENT

Another benefit that women get from the PMS myth is that it offers them an acceptable excuse to lose control. Feeling moody, irritable, the urge to withdraw, the need to communicate dissatisfaction, as well as a strong desire to put their needs first, can feel threatening to women because these behaviors are the opposite of the feminine standard. Women who attribute their negative moods to PMS describe themselves as lacking self-control if they have an emotional outburst.[28]

Why are women so afraid of losing control over their feelings? While ideal masculinity is manifested by "doing"—being active and assertive, ideal femininity is manifested by "not doing"—not being loud, coarse, intemperate, or selfish.[29] To "act like a lady" is to be polite, calm, graceful, and—above all—to care for and sacrifice for others without complaint. Achieving this ideal involves substantial self-regulation. It takes a lot of self-control to put your needs and emotions last.

Having an influence that is out of a woman's control, like PMS, is advantageous because within this paradigm her hormones are controlling her emotions without her permission. Who can be expected to fight biology? So attributing unpleasant, unladylike emotions to PMS helps a woman and others believe she hasn't willingly defied the standards of good womanhood.[30]

## A WOMAN'S ANGER CAN HURT HER

The feminine ideal extends to the workforce. At work, women's anger is perceived differently from men's anger. For men, expressing anger implies strength and capability. One study found that men who occasionally became angry at work were more likely to be accorded higher status, power, and independence by their employers, compared to men who communicated sadness.[31] For women, the story is quite different. In a series of three studies examining how people evaluate emotional expressions of professional people, study participants evaluated women who expressed anger as less competent, deserving lower wages, and rated them with lower status when compared to men who expressed anger.[32] Because their anger is unacceptable.

While women appear to experience angry thoughts just as often and strongly as men, several studies show that they express the anger differently. Women learn very early that, for them, expressing anger brings social judgment—people consider angry women to be caustic, shrill bitches. Women internalize the idea that nice women just don't get angry.[33] I know that when I was in my twenties, feeling angry made me very uncomfortable and I would invariably end up in tears—not a very good way to win an argument or make a point. As I got older, confidence in my opinions grew, but expressing angry thoughts, no matter how justified, still makes my heart race and leads me to question myself.

Another reason why women's anger is unacceptable has to do with social status. A historical look at the interactions of low- and high-status groups showed that high-status people have always been free to express anger, and low-status people are punished for showing anger or resentment; whereas they are rewarded for agreeable, submissive expressions.[34] The pretense of the "happy and content slave" helped to protect some slaves from harsh treatment. Those who resisted or complained risked even worse working conditions, beatings, and sometimes death. For much of human history, women have similarly been at the economic mercy of their fathers and husbands for survival. It has been to their advantage to be pleasant, accommodating, and self-sacrificing. Over time, women have become somewhat less economically dependent on men, however, these traits remain fundamental to the ideal of a good woman. For some, an angry woman is still a woman who is stepping above her lower status.

What do women do instead of yell or argue? One common coping strategy is to actively attempt to suppress our feelings and "keep a lid on it." We pretend that circumstances have not made us angry. If unable to quash our feelings, a secondary coping strategy is to dissociate ourselves from our anger.[35] A way to do that is to blame it on the uncontrollable hormones in PMS. This serves as a convenient way to identify an expression of anger as "not really me."

## CONTINUED BACKLASHES AGAINST EQUAL STATUS

Research suggests that it's not only traditional gender roles that are a factor in adopting the PMS label—it's also how those roles play out in the context of a heterosexual relationship. Women in lesbian relationships report premenstrual changes as less disruptive than women in heterosexual relationships.[36] How can this be true? It goes against the stereotype: the popular take on PMS would have it that two women living together would create a monthly thermonuclear meltdown with double the amount of hormonal rages.

But recent studies show that the sexual orientation of a couple alters how they interpret and deal with premenstrual changes. Male partners are more likely to believe negative, stereotypical images of PMS and are less likely to show any support or empathy to their female partner about these changes. This increases women's premenstrual distress and encourages them to feel as if they have a disorder that needs to be treated. On the other hand, lesbian partners overwhelmingly show empathetic support during a partner's premenstrual changes and interpret them as normal. This approach, in turn, makes it easier for women to use coping techniques to care for themselves, such as taking time away or avoiding conflict.[37]

Because lesbian relationships don't conform to traditional gender roles as much as heterosexual relationships do, they offer an example of what happens in an egalitarian situation. It's impossible to decide that the person with the penis must take out the garbage, change the oil in the car, and mow the lawn when there is no person with a penis. Psychologists who conduct therapy with lesbian couples find them to operate more as equals than heterosexual couples: they share power, decision-making, and household responsibilities more.[38]

This shows that there are very strong social and relational components to how premenstrual changes are experienced and interpreted. Women are not raised to think anything a girl does is weak or lame or disgusting. So these attitudes, which men typically do learn, don't come into play in a lesbian relationship. This takes away the imperative to label any mood changes a woman has, for whatever reason, as irrational and invalid.

## BLAMING BIOLOGY IS EASY, TAKING RESPONSIBILITY IS HARD

Socially, PMS makes it easy to minimize and invalidate women's concerns and opinions. And women have also reaped some benefits from wielding the PMS myth. We have been able to lose emotional control, express anger, complain, and be excused from domestic responsibilities—without losing the title of Good Woman. Women are not held responsible for these temporary trips outside of acceptable feminine behavior because PMS provides an unavoidable, biological explanation. However, these are short-term benefits that come with many costs, which I will share in detail in chapter 11. First, I'll take a look at the myths and truths about another time when women are thought to be caught in a hormonal maelstrom: during the nine months of pregnancy.

# CHAPTER 4

# The "Significantly" Impaired Preggo

The first time I was pregnant, I was amazed at how the world opened up to me with thoughtfulness and generosity. Once my belly was protruding for all to see, people were careful and gentle with me: giving me the front seat in the car, making sure I had enough to eat, carrying things for me. There was a great sense of tribal protection over me; as if a primal impulse was activated to ensure the reproduction of our species.

This also came with the belief that I wasn't able to take care of myself. The assumption extends to all pregnant women: when a coworker was pregnant and we were hit with a nor'easter snowstorm, her husband decided it was best to come pick her up. He didn't think she could make it home by herself, even though she lived close to the office and her car was already at work. Somehow, pregnancy had sucked the driving skills out of her.

Along with treating a pregnant woman as precious cargo comes the attitude that she is no longer capable; she just won't function, think, and feel like she used to. It's as if we believe that being pregnant is too much for her to bear, and that all other faculties suffer as a result.

## THE FORGETFUL, DISORGANIZED PREGNANT WOMAN

Studies show that both men and women commonly believe that cognitive abilities, like memory and problem solving, suffer because of pregnancy.

Pregnant women are portrayed in popular media as flighty and foggy. In a 2011 episode of the sitcom *How I Met Your Mother*, Lily becomes pregnant and develops "pregnancy brain." She puts her keys in the freezer and ice cubes in her pocketbook, and in a restaurant texts Robin to get directions for the way back from the bathroom. Robin tells Lily's husband, Marshall, that Lily's "brain is in a cocktail of hormones, mood swings, and nesting instincts," and that she can't be trusted to make any major life decisions.[1] Another popular show, *Modern Family*, also aired a "pregnancy brain" episode. When pregnant, Gloria is similarly scatterbrained: she puts soap in the refrigerator and butter in the shower. Her husband, Jay, refers to her as the "stupid pregnant lady" and later in the episode she tries to get out of a moving car.[2] It's clear that pregnancy has made these women loopy, forgetful, and lacking in judgment.

Pregnancy guides like the widely read, longtime bestseller *What to Expect When You Are Expecting* reinforce this by warning women of their inevitable decline by stating that hormonal changes in pregnancy make even the most organized woman a mess, unable to cope with complicated issues.[3] In recent decades, pregnancy guides have become the most influential source for establishing the "normal" pregnancy experience because we no longer live, day in and day out, among generations of women. Pregnancy feels like a mystery, so these guidebooks have become go-to sources for information.[4] And they unequivocally tell pregnant women to expect cognitive instability.

Many studies have been done to see whether this is true or not, and the results are far from conclusive: some studies find differences and some don't. A review of this research reported that of eight studies comparing the verbal recall of pregnant and nonpregnant women, three found that pregnant women could not remember verbal content as well as nonpregnant women, two studies found that pregnant women performed better, and three studies found no difference. When deficits were found in pregnant women on tasks involving verbal recall and other kinds of memory, they were by very small margins.[5] Research on the ability to stay focused and not get distracted also shows little consistent evidence of a pregnancy effect. Several studies found no difference between pregnant women and nonpregnant women.[6] When differences have been found, they have been very specific; for example, in a study on maintaining visual focus pregnant women performed worse than nonpregnant women at thirty-six weeks of pregnancy—but not at fourteen, seventeen, twenty-nine, or thirty-two weeks.[7]

Although many pregnant women say they *feel like* their abilities to remember and stay focused are impaired, research doesn't support the actual existence of a meaningful decline. As for blaming this experience on hormones, an important aspect of all the research is that it shows no consistent evidence that hormonal changes during pregnancy influence women's cognitive abilities.[8] So even if pregnancy causes small changes in memory and organizational thinking, research does not support using hormones to explain this difference.[9]

## THE WEEPING, RAGING PREGNANT WOMAN

Most people also think that pregnant women are in a constant state of emotional flux, weeping then raging—without reason. The Internet is full of websites that attest the stereotype of the deranged pregnant woman. Whether a blog on the *Huffington Post* declares "It's Official: Pregnancy Does Make You Crazy," or forum websites like *Reddit* host discussions under headings like, "Help! My pregnant wife is driving me crazy," pregnant women are presented as emotional pinballs that ricochet off one mood into another. These stories also stress that it is all out of a woman's control because of her hormones, and that the people in her life better just buckle up and deal with it.

*What to Expect When You're Expecting* features a monthly description of how a pregnant woman is likely to feel, physically and emotionally. Month after month, women are warned about "mood swings, irritability, and irrationality" because of those pesky hormones.[10] The cheekier *Girlfriends' Guide to Pregnancy* presents pregnancy "insanity" as a given, even suggesting that "feeling like you are losing your mind" is one telltale sign that there's a bun in your oven. The author recounts several violent outbursts from her own pregnancy, like grabbing the wheel from her husband while he was driving and throwing a book at his head— presenting this behavior as normal. And for the woman tempted to suspect her bad mood may actually be caused by someone or something else, the author explains that a pregnant woman simply cannot trust herself. "As convinced as you may be of your rationality and of everyone else's irrationality," she warns, "you really are not normal, and you should just accept it and allow for it."[11]

So is it true? Do women's hormones rise and jump around like popcorn in the microwave? Sort of. And do they result in extreme emotions? Yes and no—but the answer is more "no" than "yes."

## THE ACTUAL HORMONAL INFLUENCE

The major hormones involved with pregnancy are human chorionic gonadotropin (hCG), progesterone, and estrogen. These hormones are amazing chemicals that regulate a number of functions, providing for the health of the mother and the development of a fetus. What turns on a body's pregnancy switch is hGC, which initiates all kinds of processes that establish a healthy pregnancy. It encourages the empty follicle left after fertilization to produce estrogen and progesterone for the first several weeks until the placenta develops and takes over that job; it also helps keep the conditions of the uterine lining optimal for early development. In the first ten weeks of pregnancy, the hCG level escalates and doubles every day. It plateaus at about twelve weeks and then slowly reduces by 80 percent so that in the twentieth week it reaches a level that stays steady until delivery.[12]

On the other hand, progesterone and estrogen production start slowly, gradually increase throughout pregnancy, and peak with delivery at levels about ten times higher than they were in the beginning. Progesterone keeps the uterus relaxed and contributes nutrition toward sustaining the embryo. It also enables the development of the fetus and helps activate estrogen to prepare the mother's breasts for nursing. Estrogen is responsible for her increased blood volume, weight gain, enlargement of the uterus, growth of breast ducts, and relaxation of the pelvic ligaments— which makes it easier, relatively speaking, to deliver the baby.[13]

Overall, in early pregnancy there is a rapid increase in hCG, but after the twelfth week it settles down. The production of progesterone and estrogen increase substantially, but at a fairly steady rate. So does the high production of these hormones cause pregnant women to become unreasonable, emotionally erratic, and forgetful, like the hormone myth says?

Psychologists widely agree that despite the hormonal changes, pregnancy is a time of particularly *good* mental health. Pregnant women aren't any more likely to develop depression or anxiety disorders than nonpregnant women. In fact, pregnant women are actually less likely to be admitted to a psychiatric hospital, attempt suicide, or suffer from panic disorders compared to women who aren't pregnant.[14] While some women do describe their emotions during pregnancy as more fragile and changeable, the emotions expressed by the majority of pregnant women stay within the normal range of human behavior. Throughout the nine months, most women experience a stable emotional state.[15]

If it's clear that the majority of women cope well with pregnancy, what explains the emotional difficulties that a minority of women have? It's unlikely to be hormones, because if increased levels of hCG, progesterone, and estrogen truly caused emotional disorders, everyone would experience them simply because levels of hormones go up in all pregnant women.

## OTHER REASONS FOR UPSET

Psychologists have found that predictors of a women's psychological well-being during pregnancy are: her physical reaction to pregnancy, whether the pregnancy was planned, the quality of her relationship to the baby's father, and her economic status.[16] It's easy to imagine the contentedness of a financially secure woman who physically feels great during a pregnancy she planned as part of a supportive, stable relationship with the baby's father. Similarly, we can imagine the distress of a woman just barely making rent, who is vomiting daily from a pregnancy that came at a time in her life when she's struggling and occurred in a conflict-filled relationship with the baby's father.

Throughout the nine months of gestation, common concerns do come up that reflect a rational mind-set trying to cope in response to a major life transition. The extent of upset a mother-to-be feels strongly relates to the way she responds to the following changes that come with pregnancy.

### What's Happening to My Body?

Most American women don't grow up with generations of pregnant women all around them. With family size shrinking, women don't remember when their mothers or aunts were pregnant, since they were likely to have been small children at the time. Generations don't overlap anymore; a hundred years ago it wouldn't be unusual for a fifteen-year-old girl to witness the pregnancy of her forty-year-old mother and her twenty-year-old sister at the same time—as well as the pregnancies of aunts and female cousins who were likely to live nearby. Nowadays, many women step into pregnancy not knowing what physical symptoms are normal and which are medically concerning. With no idea how to interpret symptoms like nausea, spotting, fatigue, or painful breasts, it's no wonder women worry.

## What's Happening to My Appearance?

Pregnancy brings an unavoidable big belly: since all of our organs are tightly tucked in there, when a baby starts growing it inevitably sticks out. And that is the complete opposite of the Western ideal of beauty. The social pressure for women to be thin, especially in the abdominal area, is unrelenting—even during pregnancy, even though there is absolutely nothing a pregnant woman can do about it. You just can't suck in a pregnant belly. Some women feel positive about their bodily changes and see pregnancy as one of the few times in their lives when they don't have to be concerned about their weight. But other women become dissatisfied with their bodies and feel fat and ugly, especially when they hear comments about their weight from others.[17] I am a short woman and I gained thirty pounds during my first pregnancy, which is in the normal, healthy range. But apparently the extra weight made me look like a large, round ball. I was asked many times if I was having twins, when I definitely was not. Left to my own devices, I was okay about how my body had changed, but it was hard to keep that positivity up in the face of social feedback that I looked HUGE.

## What's Happening to My Marriage?

Yes, it's well-documented that satisfaction in marital relationships declines after the birth of a first child.[18] Women often expect this and even see it brewing during pregnancy. While the initial transition from having no children to being a parent is the hardest, additional children can make it even harder to maintain some kind of identity and satisfaction as a couple. Caring for a newborn is a job that goes on twenty-four hours a day and consumes huge amounts of emotional and physical energies. Pregnant women tend to worry about how they will be able to maintain their relationship with their partner in the midst of this.

## What's Happening to My Life?

Pregnancy and the birth of a baby bring massive changes to a woman's life. Professionally, she may not know how her pregnancy will be received at work or how it will impact her upward movement. If she has morning sickness and runs for the bathroom in the middle of a meeting, it doesn't appear very professional. The average age for an American woman to become a mother is at an all-time high, especially for college-educated women. It's likely that much of their identity has been invested in establishing themselves as capable and competent in the workplace, and there's nothing like a first baby to strip away those competent feelings. She may worry about how she will cover her bills if her company doesn't provide paid maternity leave, as most US companies don't. And even if her partner says that he is committed to sharing in the tasks of caring for the baby, she may wonder whether it will really work out that way. Or will he, like so many men, revert to more traditional gender roles when the baby comes?

These challenges can feel disruptive and do affect a woman's mood. Still, there is so much evidence that pregnant women's psychological states and mental abilities stay in the normal range. So why do we believe the hormone myth more, which says the opposite is true? A look at the establishment of the "baby brain" myth reveals a lot.

## FLAWED SCIENCE AND BAD REPORTING STRIKE AGAIN

A 2014 article in *The Daily Telegraph* defines the now-popular concept of *baby brain* as a "pregnancy-induced fog," in which many women claim to "become more forgetful during pregnancy, oversensitive, and less able to focus on logical tasks."[19] This experience was thoroughly legitimized by the profoundly inaccurate reporting of flawed research by popular news outlets. Scholar Nicole Hurt uses rhetorical studies, feminist theory, and media coverage of health research to understand how texts construct social norms and behavior. She identified the widespread and harmful effects of the misrepresentation of one study, which solidified our belief in the existence of baby brain.[20]

"A Review of the Impact of Pregnancy on Memory Function" was published in 2007. The rationale for the review was the observation that, even though between 50 and 80 percent of pregnant women *report* a decline in their cognitive abilities during pregnancy, the research measuring women's *actual* cognitive abilities while pregnant produce very mixed results, sometimes finding differences and sometimes not. Drawing on studies that show people, in general, aren't very good at estimating their cognitive abilities, the researchers set out to examine the most recent studies on pregnant women's cognitive abilities to reach an overall conclusion about how one variable influences another variable. They were careful to include only the methodologically stronger studies that included a control group of nonpregnant women as they examined research on the influence of pregnancy on seven different types of memory.[21]

When researchers statistically measure the relationship of one variable to another, their calculations produce a correlation, labeled as an "r value." In psychology, an r value of 0.1 is considered a small effect, 0.3 has a medium effect, and 0.5 and up indicates a large effect.[22] The researchers calculated average r values to measure the effect of pregnancy on seven different types of memory. The results ranged from 0.09—with pregnant women performing marginally better than nonpregnant ones; to -0.26—showing that pregnant women performed slightly worse than nonpregnant women. The overall r value for the effect of pregnancy on all seven types of memory was -0.12. What this means is that pregnancy has a very small negative effect on memory. It's not an open question that the results convey a very small effect—psychologists have used these guidelines to understand study data for decades.

However, the authors of this study didn't describe the results of their review that way. Instead, they wrote, "The results indicate that pregnant women are *significantly* impaired on some, but not all, measures of memory." I added the italics to emphasize the word "significantly," because the use of that word is essential to the interpretation of data. It is important to know whether the correlation found is "statistically significant," which indicates at least 95-percent confidence that the differences found between groups reflect actual differences, rather than those produced by chance. While the overall effect of pregnancy on memory was statistically significant, that doesn't mean the difference is "significant" in the way that word is used in common conversation. Commonly used, it implies something meaningful or noteworthy or substantial. Despite the difference in uses of this word, the authors used it to imply the common meaning. Their results described a significant impairment and they suggested that their findings show the need to research the causes and "functional consequences of pregnancy-related memory difficulties."

What difficulties? This review found that when they do exist, difficulties with memory while pregnant are very small. Therefore, most would agree that studying why these very small differences exist would not explain much about the psychological experience of pregnancy. The study's conclusion was flawed.

## A CASE OF MISTAKEN FACT

The popular press loves running stories that frame women's mental states as biologically based. And did they ever love this one. The review was reported by television stations, websites, and newspapers across the United States and the world, including in England, India, Australia, Sudan, and New Zealand. Newspapers took the word "significant" and ran with it. They described the study as revealing that "pregnant women are significantly impaired," or that they are "considerably impaired," and that pregnancy causes "considerable memory loss."

Not only was the result presented as much more powerful than it actually was, it was presented as a final confirmation that baby brain really does exist. Headlines ran: "Baby Brain's Not Myth," "Baby Brain Myth Becomes a Reality," and the definitive "Pregnancy Does Cause Memory Loss." The press took the researchers' misrepresentation of data one step further, confusing data, language, and fact to produce the most sensational story possible. Effectively putting the final screw in the public's perception of the reality of the forgetful pregnant woman, the press outright misreported an important statistic presented in the review. At the opening of their study report, the psychologists stated that previous studies indicated that between 50 and 80 percent of pregnant women *report* a decline in their cognitive abilities, with the further caveat that people are shown to be not very good at evaluating their own cognitive abilities. But the media coverage mistakenly informed the public that the study found an *actual decline* in the cognitive abilities of 50 to 80 percent of pregnant women—and furthermore presented the statistic as if it were the result of their review and not the preamble.

These numbers sound convincing—even though they are completely inaccurate. Belief in baby brain as a real phenomenon was cemented in popular culture because we thought science had proved it. Since then, additional studies have attempted to overcome the myth. But the storyline is now too tight to easily unravel.

## BLAMING BABY BRAIN

When people believe that pregnant women are overemotional and flighty because of their hormones, it becomes easy to decide that their distresses and complaints can be simply ignored. The perceptions are that, if behavior is caused by biology, there is no avoiding it and no need to take it seriously. In the same way women can be cut down by the PMS label, when pregnant women's thoughts, opinions, and actions get blamed on overactive hormones, they become devalued and lose credibility as rational human beings. In relationships and the workplace, their status is diminished.

When a pregnant woman becomes angry or forgetful, calling it baby brain also delegitimizes the actual cause. It excuses others from having to deal with situational issues she may be facing, such as an inflexible corporate culture that makes being pregnant miserable or doing the majority of the work to prepare for the baby. It may seem like all a pregnant woman has to do is gestate, but anyone who has been a mother-to-be knows there is plenty to do: educating ourselves on pregnancy and newborn care, arranging for childcare after maternity leave, negotiating how to reintegrate work after the baby comes, and buying all the myriad products needed. Even nowadays, it is still most likely that these responsibilities will be the woman's, even though she and her husband probably work similar hours. The hormone myth gives a firm basis for the idea that a woman's concerns are "all in her head"—and therefore there is no point of working toward, or even supporting, positive change. Because these signs that our social structures still have a very gendered nature simply gets deflected.[23]

The many physical and social adjustments that pregnant women make during this transitional time do more to inspire strong emotional responses than hormones. But expectations color everyone's interpretation of their behavior. Authorities on all levels, from websites to news outlets, inaccurately reinforce the perception that hormones make women emotionally erratic and cognitively impaired—directly in the face of substantial scientific and experiential evidence that for most women, this is not the case. Pregnant women's mental health is not only similar to nonpregnant women, they even appear to have some advantages.[24]

Cultural myths wield tremendous power, so just as an angry woman one week before her period will be more likely to attribute her mood to PMS, a pregnant woman is more likely to attribute an emotional outburst or forgetful moment to elevated hormones—even though it's much more probable that it was caused by feelings of overwhelm and stress. But by dismissing her experience, the problems that are upsetting her persist. Now that you can see the myth, let's explore how it is maintained, as the employment, medical care, and social interactions of pregnant women are bound up in it.

# CHAPTER 5

# A Pregnant Body
# Rules a Woman

Women's reproductive functions are generally thought to be so animalistic and unrefined that any evidence of them has historically been kept private. This view is profoundly evident in the way pregnancy was hidden. From medieval through early twentieth centuries, middle- and upper-class sensibilities required a pregnant woman who was showing to refrain from being in public. Pregnancy was not a subject for polite conversation—a woman was not pregnant, she was in "a delicate condition" or "the family way"—basically in a shameful state because she was being ruled by her body.

As a species, we tend to relish a sense of superiority because rationality allows us to rise above our bodies. To say that people are "acting like animals" is to say they are behaving basely, purely from instinct and biological drive—without the thoughtful reflectiveness and refinement that humans ideally display. Cultural norms about sex, eating, and taking care of bodily functions exist to raise us above nature, providing the sense of having a higher purpose in the universe than animals do.[1] Consistently, women's personalities and behaviors have been associated with the body, while men's have been associated with the mind. People continue to see women as more intuitive, emotional, and irrational than men—a way of thinking that has had a profound influence on the status and treatment of women because it takes us further away from the human ideal of rationality and mentally driven responses.[2]

So perpetuating the myth that rising hormones make pregnant women irrational and incompetent hurts women because it positions them closer to a biologically-driven, animal-like image. This deeply rooted connection between women and the body has, culturally, led us to perceive pregnancy as a time when a woman's body rules over her rationality and therefore, we need to approach pregnancy as an illness.

## THE MEDICALIZATION OF PREGNANCY

In the centuries before there were physicians, women were the healers who cared for other women when sick, tended them throughout their pregnancies, and delivered their babies. The local wisewoman or midwife treated her patients using herbs, remedies, and knowledge that had been passed down over the generations. This knowledge was shared among women in an open network of collegiality.[3]

The shift away from seeing pregnancy as a normal bodily process to thinking of it as an illness that requires medical treatment began in the early 1900s. Obstetrics as a medical specialty took hold then, and continues today, with an ever-increasing number of interventions and tests.[4] This male-dominated medical profession was a result of the scientific revolution, during which it was determined that science—not folklore—was the best basis for medical care. For these new male doctors, the best way to promote their services was to denigrate the folk wisdom of midwives and to ultimately make it illegal for them to practice medicine. One way that doctors distinguished themselves from female healers was to practice active medicine, also known as "heroic medicine." In the early days of the medical profession, doctors prescribed treatments with dramatic effects, such as bloodletting and purgatives—even though they made people sicker, not better.[5]

This same mentality of active medicine inspired the medicalization of normal bodily processes like pregnancy. To justify their superiority over the decidedly less interventionist approach of midwives, doctors reconceived pregnancy as a sickness that could only be managed with the expertise of a man of science. A doctor doesn't make any money without sick people to treat and so, with pregnancy categorized as a threatening condition to be managed, a continuous supply of "sick" people was created.

An especially harmful result of this mentality is that it changed women's statuses as healers for each other. Pregnancy and childbirth were previously processes of female cooperation: the midwife and close female relatives taught a woman what to expect along the way, how to manage events, and then helped manage her household in late pregnancy and early postpartum. When obstetricians took over, these men became the authority and the woman was required to take the role of unquestioning subordinate.[6] A woman's competence, to know her body and how to take care of it, was no longer trusted. This model of doctor–patient relationships—particularly male doctor to female patient—laid the groundwork for the medical field to label women's hormones as the source of so much physical and emotional infirmity. The understanding was that, while reproductive processes are animalistic and have their own rhythm, only the doctor understands them for the danger they pose—and can tame them.

Of course, there have been some undeniable health benefits to the increased use of medical technology, such as the reduction of maternal death because of *placenta previa*—which is when the placenta covers the cervix, and *ectopic pregnancy*—when a fertilized egg implants in a fallopian tube rather than the uterus.[7] However, the medicalization of pregnancy has also brought excessive medical interventions with little proven benefit. Like the useless and sometimes expensive "cures" for PMS, the hormone myth's portrayal of the female body as defective and in need of constant monitoring has led to practices such as performing excessive numbers of ultrasound screenings.

## "JUST A QUICK PEEK TO BE SURE EVERYTHING'S OKAY"

When my friends and I were going through our pregnancies in the 1990s, getting the ultrasound was exciting—even if we could barely see our baby's shape in the midst of dots. These days, 3D ultrasounds make the existence of a baby within a pregnant woman's stomach evermore real and tangible. For many, this marks the beginning of the love affair with their babies. This initial, diagnostic ultrasound provides medical benefits that include accurate dating of the pregnancy, identification of the exact location of the pregnancy to be sure it's not ectopic, proving viability, recognizing multiple pregnancies, and locating the placenta.[8]

In the initial decades after this technology was developed, the norm was to perform one to two ultrasound screenings before delivery for all low-risk pregnancies—and that remains the standard today.[9] But in practice, something changed along the way. Nowadays, women are getting many more ultrasounds with very little, if any, medical cause. In 2013, doctors performed an average of four to five ultrasound screenings per pregnancy,[10] despite evidence that doing so provides no additional health benefits for the baby or mother.[11]

Yes, women enjoy seeing their baby in utero, but there are serious risks to excessive screening. Every time an ultrasound is done, there is a risk of a false positive that reports abnormalities that are not there. This can trigger unnecessary additional testing and, in the worst-case scenario, the termination of a pregnancy due to a misperception of an abnormality. Another risk is reporting errors, such as inaccurate dating of the pregnancy or failure to document important findings. Basically, the more times a test is performed, the more times these mistakes can happen.[12] The FDA has also warned that, although there is no current evidence that excessive ultrasounds harm a fetus, the fact that the procedure can create vibrations and heating of fetal tissue means it should not be "regarded as completely innocuous."[13]

So why are doctors doing so many ultrasounds? There are several reasons. Some obstetricians have become very defensive in the way they practice medicine, believing the more tests the better, because of the fear of getting sued.[14] Ob-gyns pay astronomical malpractice insurance rates because, among all specialties, they have one of the highest risks of being sued by patients. As a result, they are particularly diligent in testing to provide some protection if there should be a negative outcome. Performing ultrasounds also makes money: once a physician has invested in a machine for the office, it has to be paid off; when it is, it produces considerable revenue. Also, in a day and age when insurance companies provide lower and lower payments to doctors for patient contact, income from doing tests can help make up for that loss. And finally, justification for excessive screening comes from the central tenet of the hormone myth: that all female reproductive functions are dangerous illnesses that can't happen successfully without continuous medical evaluation. Thinking of pregnancy as a disrupting health challenge makes excessive evaluation through ultrasounds seem appropriate.

As you can see, not one of these motivations has anything to do with a woman's health or the health of her baby.

## POLICING PREGNANT BODIES

The suspicion of the reproductive process inherent in the hormone myth has fueled the idea that pregnancy is a sickness, which has led to another consequence of medicalizing it: the surveillance of pregnant women. The understanding is that a pregnant body is permanently at risk of danger, requiring a woman's self-surveillance and the surveillance of her physician—as well as anyone in her orbit. The combination of extensive medical monitoring throughout pregnancy, unending pregnancy guide warnings like "Don't eat soft cheese!," and the anxiety-provoking information on the Internet has created a cultural perception that there is always something to worry about. And the best way a woman can display that she is a good mother-to-be is to worry about everything, all the time.[15]

### You Better Not Do This, That, and the Other Thing

I remember participating in the "I'm-more-careful-than-you Olympics" when I was pregnant the same time a friend was. When I noticed her drinking hot chocolate, I said, "Did you know? There's a lot of caffeine in chocolate." When she noticed me eating a ham sandwich, she said, "I would never eat cold cuts. The nitrates are bad for the baby." In retrospect, it was ridiculous. We were healthy women who didn't drink or smoke and ate quite nutritiously—who eventually did have perfectly healthy babies. And it was extremely likely that we would. But what was clear to us was that our attention to risk was required, no matter how minute.

Many well-known "don'ts" are based on theoretical risks, with little or no evidence to back them up. For example, pregnant women have been told not to eat sushi for fear of parasites. But there is actually very little risk. The fish used for sushi is unlikely to have parasites and it is flash-frozen, killing the few parasites that may exist. The risk of food poisoning from eating sushi is one in two-million servings, whereas the risk of food poisoning from eating chicken is one in 25,000 servings.[16] But we've never been advised to restrict eating chicken while pregnant, which shows that these "don'ts" can be nonsensical.

Debunking them is an aside; maybe it's not such a big deal that pregnant women don't eat sushi when they really could. Better to be on the safe side, right? The problem I'm pointing to is that this constant monitoring, which women are supposed to do, has become a moral responsibility. It implies that a woman can have total control over her baby's health and safe delivery if she just does everything right. When the reality is: she can't control everything about her environment; even when she can, she may be worrying about the wrong things; and sometimes, without a knowable medical explanation, pregnancies don't go well. In this situation, the hormone myth hurts women because its assumption that women's reproductive processes are inherently illnesses that require medical treatment erroneously creates the expectation that this treatment is infallible, and it is therefore within each woman's power to produce a perfect pregnancy if she will only follow all the rules—both reasonable and not reasonable.

## You Actually Should Have...

The exaggeration and misperception of risk also keeps pregnant women from *doing* things that would improve their health.[17] Doctors strongly urge pregnant women to be vaccinated for the flu, however, only 15 percent comply. There is solid evidence that maternal flu vaccination causes no negative outcomes for the fetus. But because women mistakenly suspect there is a risk, they put themselves at higher risk of contracting the flu—which is more likely to cause severe illness in pregnant women than nonpregnant women, and can cause preterm labor and delivery.[18]

Some women with severe asthma stop using their medication because they are worried about harm to the fetus. However, uncontrolled asthma is associated with dangerous repercussions for both the mother and the fetus, like early miscarriage, uterine hemorrhage, prematurity, and low birthweight. Studies show that women with well-controlled asthma have babies that are just as healthy as women without asthma. Still, the presumption of ever-present danger keeps some women from using medication that is proven to be beneficial.[19]

The idea that pregnancy creates a such a fragile state works against women and ironically keeps them from doing things that will actually improve their health and the health of the baby.

## You Should Find Out If...

The fear of any risk during pregnancy has also created a culture that expects women to test fetuses for possible genetic problems. At first this may seem like a practice that gives women more information and control over their pregnancy, but the control to do what? One of the most common prenatal tests detects chromosomal disorders like Down syndrome, and if the genetic anomalies associated with a disorder are found, a woman has only two choices: abort the fetus or deliver a disabled child. There is no treatment available.

The expectation of constant surveillance to ensure the production of a perfect baby can make it socially unacceptable for a woman to have a baby with a disability. Medical professionals, family, and friends may blame the woman for allowing this child to be born, and therefore be less likely to provide support.[20] A friend of mine had her first baby after thirty-five, the usual age at which testing for Down syndrome becomes routine because of the increased risk. She declined the test, because she was okay with the possibility of raising a child with this disorder. Her doctor was incredulous, finding it inconceivable that she was willing to take this risk, and pressured her to be tested. The culture of surveillance and prenatal testing worked to curtail her autonomy, rather than to truly give her choices. It was only with her resistance to this culture that she achieved true autonomy.

The great majority of pregnancies brought to term produce healthy babies. Yet still, the hormone myth feeds on the idea that pregnancy is among the dangerous functions that women's bodies perform. So with everyone assuming that pregnancy is a time rife with risk and that it requires constant vigilance to produce a perfect child, constant worrying seems like the only responsible thing to do. And it turns out that with pregnancy, you can worry yourself and your baby sick.

## WHAT REALLY HAPPENS WHEN PREGNANT WOMEN WORRY

The reality is that worry itself is the true threat. We all experience some level of stress in our daily lives, but stress overload during pregnancy is bad for women and their babies. Research indicates that feeling stressed during pregnancy is very common: up to 78 percent of pregnant women experience low to moderate stress[21] and estimates for acute stress range from 6 to 27 percent. For women, acute and chronically elevated stress during pregnancy is related to feelings of anxiety and depression[22] and a higher rate of miscarriage.[23] It is also associated with higher incidences of low birthweight, preterm birth, and congenital defects of the fetus.[24]

After delivery, the child of a mother who experienced acute or chronic stress during pregnancy is at a higher risk for poor physical and mental outcomes. There is convincing research that shows a mother's stress-overload during pregnancy is associated with her infant's emotional and behavioral problems, lower childhood IQ, and slightly higher risk for symptoms of ADHD. Physically, children are more likely to suffer from infections, insulin resistance, and a variety of diseases.[25]

Feeling stressed has a very real impact on a pregnant woman's health and that of her baby—and the hypermedicalized approach to pregnancy that I have described throughout this chapter compounds the harming experiences of worry and stress.

# A RETURN TO PERCEIVING REPRODUCTION AS NATURAL

Are there other ways to think about, and care for, pregnant women that cause less stress and therefore less harm? One subculture that sees repro-duction as a natural process in need of little intervention is the midwifery model, which offers some compelling—and substantial—differences from the medicalized and risk-oriented model of modern obstetrics.[26] A certi-fied midwife and also a nurse-midwife will initiate care with the assump-tion that every woman's body is capable of maintaining a healthy pregnancy. There is continuity when a midwife provides prenatal care, as the pregnant woman sees the same midwife for every visit. The relation-ship that results makes it more likely that the pregnant woman is seen as whole person, rather than a list of risks to manage. A midwifes generally charges one fee for prenatal care and the delivery, resulting in visits that aren't as time-limited as doctor appointments, which are scheduled so the most patients can be seen in as short a time span as possible. This makes it possible for the midwife to address a woman's concerns about her preg-nancy, delivery, and postpartum life as they come up, as well as to teach her about future issues, like breastfeeding and caring for a newborn. This all creates a different environment for a pregnant woman, as it trusts her body's capability and facilitates the transition from mother-to-be to mother with no hysteria or extreme focus on risk.

Can this be safe for women? It already is. A thorough review of thirteen randomized controlled studies comparing more than 16,000 women who received care from a midwife or an obstetrician found no differences in their safety. In fact, women who were under a midwife's care, prenatally and for delivery, were less likely to miscarry before twenty-four weeks and also less likely to have a preterm birth.[27] Women who did develop high-risk pregnancies, with issues like placenta previa or gestational diabetes, were referred to a physician's care.

Yet only 9 percent of American women get their prenatal and delivery care from a midwife.[28] Why not more? Because the power of the hormone myth maintains the imperative that all reproductive events need to be exhaustively managed. If a woman doesn't utilize the medical system at its highest level, the myth says she is irresponsible—despite some very convincing science that tells us otherwise.

## THE MANY STIGMAS OF SHOWING AT WORK

In terms of health care, thinking of pregnancy as a sickness evokes responses of surveillance and worry, and in the workplace it conveys an aura of delicate femininity and incompetence. I'm sure you've either seen, or been, a pregnant woman at work—which is no surprise since about 75 percent of women will be employed while pregnant.[29] Unfortunately, it does change the way employers and colleagues think about a woman—and not for the better. Our cultural belief in the emotional instability and cognitive deficit of pregnant women lead to discriminations against them in the workplace that are tangible. The hormone myth promotes the stereotype of pregnant women as overemotional, which many believe is incompatible with competent leadership.[30] Psychologists and business analysts have reported the following ways in which pregnancy is a stigma that women must negotiate at work.[31]

### The Height of Femininity Bombs at Work

The unavoidable, visual evidence of pregnancy, a protruding belly, invokes the stereotype of a traditional female and a traditional role. What could be more emblematic of womanhood than a pregnant female? She must be nurturing, warm, emotional, and committed to home and family. Her impending motherhood calls forth one of the central qualities of a good woman—that she is always available, emotionally and physically, to her family.[32]

These qualities are problematic in the context of the workplace because the ideal employee is completely different: always available, not to her family, but to her employer. She doesn't bring family concerns or other outside matters to work and demonstrates her commitment to the company by cheerfully working countless hours.[33] And especially in management positions, she must have characteristics that reflect traditional male stereotypes, such as being active, confident, rational, and assertive.[34] The inevitable conflict between these ideals creates irreconcilable conditions for her employer, boss, and colleagues to navigate within.

## Conflicted Feelings Surface in Others

Thinking about an employee in entirely feminine terms renders her unfit to work in any setting outside the home. When people discern a lack of fit between a person's perceived ability and job requirements, their expectations of failure increase.[35] A pregnant woman in the workplace may also activate others' conflicted feelings about whether mothers should work at all. Despite the facts that maintaining a middle-class lifestyle most commonly requires the paid labor of both spouses, that poor mothers have always worked, and that the majority of mothers currently are employed, we still hear about "mommy wars" and the debate over whether mothers should leave their children to work or not. Those in the office who subscribe to traditional gender roles may judge a working mother-to-be harshly because she represents a violation of mother-as-homemaker role.[36]

## "She Won't Come Back"

At the same time, colleagues may be resentful because they assume a pregnant woman won't return to work after the birth of the baby.[37] In reality, about 75 percent of pregnant women return to their jobs,[38] but coworkers and supervisors commonly believe they won't.[39] This can make them feel that discrimination against pregnant workers is legitimate. The result is that being committed to her job doesn't actually do anything for a pregnant woman—as her boss and colleagues simply won't believe her.

This is beyond unfair. What does a woman have to do to convince people that she is coming back? Take out an ad? Perform hypnosis? Prejudice and outright discrimination thrive because people can't get the idea that pregnant women are the same competent and dedicated employees they were before they got pregnant.

## Continually Questioned Competence

Studies examining the treatment of pregnant women in the workplace have found that interviewers treat pregnant women applying for a job more rudely than nonpregnant women, especially if they are applying for a traditionally perceived male job, like engineer or auto mechanic.[40] Throughout the whole employment experience, from interviewing to evaluating to firing, coworkers and supervisors treat pregnant women differently and their competence is doubted. Two different studies had participants watch videos of working women and evaluate them. The pregnant women were evaluated as less capable and less appropriate for promotion.[41] Study participants were also less likely to recommend hiring a pregnant woman than a nonpregnant woman.[42]

# THE HORMONE MYTH FUELS ILLEGAL DISCRIMINATION PRACTICES

Just seeing a woman with a pregnant belly seems to bring on feelings and actions that hurt women at work—and that are illegal under United States employment discrimination laws. One recent example is the case of Mallory Barker, an arts and crafts instructor at a Wisconsin private school. Barker had been employed at the school without incident for two months, but two days after her boss found out she was pregnant, she received a voicemail telling her she was being let go because it "just wasn't working out."[43] She submitted a complaint to the Equal Employment Opportunity Commission (EEOC), which sued the school for pregnancy discrimination on her behalf. In March 2013, the presiding judge ruled that Barker had been discriminated against, and that the school owed her back pay. The school also agreed to train its employees, managers, and supervisors in employee rights, as well as how to avoid pregnancy discrimination.[44]

EEOC statistics confirm that discrimination due to pregnancy is not unusual. Lawsuits are filed throughout many industries, including education, social services, manufacturing, legal, and real estate, and by women in high- and low-status positions. Violations include "refusing to hire, failing to promote, demoting, or firing pregnant workers after learning they are pregnant" and retaliating against anyone who complains about pregnancy discrimination.[45]

This kind of discrimination, whether reported or not, contributes to making gender-based income inequality so persistent. It's not because women don't do the same work as men, but because of the myth that they can't do the same work due to their ability to reproduce.

# PRETENDING NO ACCOMMODATION IS NEEDED

Pregnant women know how pregnancy can hurt their careers. Many hesitate to inform employers and colleagues of a pregnancy because they fear being seen as incompetent or uncommitted. In interviews with women who had worked during pregnancy, 80 percent saw their pregnancies as a potential threat to their professional image.

A common strategy they reported using to manage their image was to maintain the same level of hours and output, which was not a problem for women with an "easy pregnancy" but required more effort for those dealing with morning sickness or exhaustion. They also purposely refrained from asking coworkers or supervisors for any special accommodations. These women minimized the amount of time missed for doctor visits, refused to ask for help, declined all offers of help, and accepted assignments involving travel—even when it was difficult. Trudging through airports and being wedged into an airplane seat for hours can be trying for the fittest of people, but pregnant women may do this while getting nauseous or carrying an extra twenty pounds around. Some women reported working even harder than usual to emphasize their dedication, and a small minority even decided to take shorter maternity leaves than was permitted. In a couple of extreme cases, women chose not to follow their doctors' orders to cut back on work, for fear of a poor evaluation or losing their job.[46]

What a shame for all of this to be necessary. Should work be a nine-month probationary period in which the image of a dedicated, productive, and completely unchanged employee is tested? There is a big difference between someone who takes time to go to the doctor once a month and turns down travel assignment and someone who is incompetent and unable to do her job. But there is an all-or-nothing mentality here, and women are so afraid of activating the pregnancy stigma that they are going to great lengths to avoid it. And, in the process, they are adding considerable, harmful stress to their pregnancies.

## DEVELOPING WORK LIFE BEFORE FAMILY LIFE

When women see pregnancy as something that threatens their professional image and puts obstacles in their career path, they delay childbearing. The rate of women who have their first child between the ages of thirty-five and forty-four has substantially increased in recent years, especially for college-educated women.[47] Delaying childbirth until this time allows women to establish thriving careers and brings an annual increase in earnings of 9 percent *for every year* motherhood is delayed.[48] It helps women avoid, or at least stave off, pregnancy discrimination and "the motherhood penalty," a well-documented phenomenon in which women without children earn higher wages and have higher wage growth compared to women with children.[49]

But there are very real medical risks to substantially delaying motherhood. Compared to women who conceive in their twenties, women who conceive in their late-thirties have a higher risk of miscarriage and are more likely to have chronic medical conditions that can create complications during pregnancy, like high blood pressure. Fertility rates drop after the early thirties, increasing the need for reproductive assistance to become pregnant—which has a higher chance of producing multiple births that bring additional health risks to the mother.[50]

# BOXING WOMEN IN

Women would be better off if they could: decide when they want to throw their energies into their career and when they want to have children, timing things so that it all makes sense and makes them happy; be professionally assessed based on their actual work without getting penalized for imagined incompetence; and take appropriate care of themselves while pregnant without fearing it will cost them a job, promotion, or raise. But the persistent and prevailing hormone myth reinforces the idea that pregnancy must change women in ways that threaten their competence, emotional stability, and even their thinking. What is the result of this cultural tradition of preconceived notions? That women get boxed in. Making decisions about family and work becomes a claustrophobic choice of "What part of my life is going to suffer most?" rather than following the many possible paths that circumstances and growth bring. This is not progress, it's a straitjacket with no easy way out. All of the circumstances I described in this chapter create tremendous stress and feelings of overwhelm within pregnant women, and may indeed be factors that contribute to moodiness and disturbance. The truth is that it is more a social, economic, and relational issue than it is a hormonal one.

Life does change after pregnancy and, as the next chapter will also show, there are more circumstances that can contribute to mental health issues in a woman after the baby is born than her hormones.

# CHAPTER 6

# The Media's Perfect Postpartum Storm

Every minute of every day, somewhere, a woman gives birth to a baby. It is a common everyday occurrence, and for most people it is a momentous occasion. The prospect of bringing a new life safely into this world is wondrous and inspires feelings of awe, excitement, and gratitude. We don't even need to know a woman personally to feel this; when the Duchess of Cambridge, Kate Middleton, delivered her first child with Prince William, I felt the specialness of the occasion and was truly happy for them. From royalty to the neighbor next door, the birth of a baby is something we celebrate with joy.

What we can't fully anticipate is what happens when that baby comes home. The addition of a child, especially a first one, brings tumultuous change to a woman's daily life. Sleep deprivation? Check. Feedings that refuse to be scheduled? Check. Mountains of laundry with spit-up? Double check. Not changing out of pajamas until four o'clock in the afternoon? Check again. Figuring out how to care for a newborn and still maintain some sense of self is a challenge every new mother has to figure out.

Most women eventually adjust, find ways to bring some predictability to their days, and manage the multitude of new responsibilities facing them. But some women struggle. Many studies indicate that there is an increased risk of mood disorders after childbirth.[1] Some women get the baby blues and cry for no reason during the days after delivery. And some become despondent to the point that getting out of bed is a challenge—an experience known as postpartum depression, which is a very real phenomenon.

Unfortunately, if you read about postpartum depression in magazine or newspaper articles or on health websites, it is challenging to sift through the myths and biases to find accurate information. The media has made some incorrect conclusions about postpartum depression that they can't let go of, for reasons that range from carelessness to a love of sensationalism—no matter how wrong they get the story. And many of these conclusions are steeped in the assumptions at the core of the hormone myth.

## WE DON'T NEED TO FIX THE WORLD, YOU JUST NEED TO FIX YOU

If after having a baby you experience sadness and depression rather than being utterly delighted and radiant, our culture thinks something is wrong with you and that you need to fix yourself. You need to see your doctor. You need to get help. While of course it makes sense for depressed mothers to get help, inherent in these exhortations is that the problem is you; it doesn't have anything to do with other people, social expectations, or institutions that dictate the options we have in the way we live. In one of the earliest articles about postpartum depression to appear in a popular magazine, a 1960 edition of *Good Housekeeping* tells readers that if after having a baby a "woman goes into an apparently causeless state of depression" she should see her doctor for tranquilizers or other medications.[2] There is no mention of things like social isolation or the role her husband plays. Today, when looking up how to prevent postpartum depression on WebMD, you are advised to "ask for help from others so you can get as much sleep, healthy food, exercise, and overall support as possible," but it doesn't say how you are supposed to get that help or why it might be difficult to get.[3]

We live in the twenty-first century, but the birth of a baby seems to activate a 1950s sensibility. Many couples fall into more traditional gender roles, even if they had a fairly egalitarian marriage before the baby. For example, many women hear things like, "Since you're home, do we really need to still pay a cleaning woman?" Articles and websites say nothing about how unfair it feels when a woman shoulders the bulk of the burden of childcare and household responsibilities. Nor do they suggest that, if a woman is overwhelmed, her husband might possibly take a paternity leave so she can go back to work.[4]

Plus, American workplaces still operate under the assumption that employees are men. Few companies offer paid maternity leave, and hardly anyone can afford to take three months of unpaid leave. Think of the stress this brings if a woman wants to care for her new baby but the economic reality makes it impossible. Do these articles or websites offer advice about how to lobby a senator to pass laws that change these policies, or how to change corporate culture? Never. They advise women that it is imperative to fix themselves by seeking treatment with medications and therapy.

## THE HORMONE ASSUMPTION

The most common thing articles and websites convey is that a woman who is sad after having a baby should fix her hormones. This is because many presume that the rapid decline of reproductive hormones after childbirth causes postpartum depression. Mayo Clinic's website tells women: "After childbirth, a dramatic drop in hormones (estrogen and progesterone) in your body may contribute to postpartum depression."[5] In a story about celebrities who've had postpartum depression, *Parents* magazine quoted actress Courtney Cox as saying she had been told by her doctor that she developed postpartum depression because "her hormones had been pummeled."[6]

This seems logical and fits into our cultural understanding of women's emotions as biologically based. It echoes the central tenet of the hormone myth: that women's reproductive processes are really illnesses that wreak havoc with women's emotions and need to be treated. However, as I will discuss more in the next chapter, while hormones play a role in the fleeting postpartum blues that only last one week, their role in causing serious postpartum mood disorders is negligible. Thorough reviews of the studies on this in the past twenty years fail to show a clear link between changes in reproductive hormones and the occurrence of postpartum depression. While it appears that the mental health of a small minority of women is threatened by hormonal change, this is not the case for the great majority of women. In fact, most studies find that hormone changes have no role in developing postpartum depression when it does occur.[7]

I know that this may be the opposite of everything you've heard about postpartum depression, but the science is clear: there are several reasons why women develop postpartum depression, but changes in hormones isn't one of them.

# ALL THE WAYS THE MEDIA GETS IT WRONG

Magazines and websites describe postpartum depression by listing symptoms, treatments, and statistics on how commonly women experience it. They make this seem straightforward, but there actually isn't just one type of postpartum mood disorder, there are three. The first is *postpartum blues*, which last just a few days after childbirth and involves mood swings and sensitivity. The second is *postpartum depression*, which lasts for two weeks or longer and involves the same symptoms as major depression diagnosed in nonmothers: sadness, hopelessness, fatigue, and an inability to enjoy things that used to generate happy feelings. And the third is *postpartum psychosis*, which is an extremely rare but very serious disorder with which a woman experiences hallucinations and delusions. Here are the other things that the media gets wrong.

## Problems with Statistics About Who Gets It

When researchers examined articles on postpartum mood disorders published in popular magazines like *Parents* magazine, *Time*, and *Ladies' Home Journal* from 1952 to 2004, they found routine confusion in descriptions of the symptoms of each disorder and how common the disorders are.[8] In the 2016 story in *Parents* magazine about celebrities, readers were told: "It's estimated that up to 25 percent will have some form of more serious postpartum depression." The reality is that only about 10 percent of women experience an episode of major depression after childbirth.[9] *Working Mother* magazine polled 500 women and found that 91 percent had "felt depressed at some time in the year after having their baby," and presented this percentage as a meaningful number.[10] But it's not meaningful because they portrayed "feeling depressed" as the same as having a major depressive episode. It's not the same at all. Everyone feels depressed sometimes, and it doesn't reflect a mental illness in need of treatment. The author was just caught up in the hormone myth, which says that childbirth makes women mentally ill.

## Confusion About Onset

Some magazines are ready to identify any time a woman feels depressed as postpartum depression. The same *Working Mother* article told readers that "postpartum depression can wallop you years after" you have the baby. In general, psychologists identify a woman's depressive episode as having a "postpartum onset" if it occurs within one year after delivery—and the official diagnosis criteria include only an onset of four weeks after delivery. The British newspaper the *Daily Mail*, which has a wide online readership in the United States, ran a story in 2014 with a bizarre headline: "Baby blues more likely FOUR years after birth: First year of motherhood is not lowest point, research reveals." First of all, post-partum blues or "baby blues" can only happen during the first week after childbirth. Second, if a woman has depressive symptoms four years after her child was born, it's unlikely that it has anything to do with birthing.

## Blending Depression with Psychosis

Perhaps the most dangerous way that the media fails at providing accurate information is that it often mixes up the symptoms of postpartum depression with postpartum psychosis. These are two very different disorders. Remember, postpartum depression involves feeling sad, hopeless, a lack of pleasure, and fatigue; the same as depression experienced by people who haven't just had a baby. Postpartum psychosis is an extremely rare condition that only one in one-thousand women experience, with which a woman has a psychotic break with reality: she hallucinates, has delusions, and may have thoughts of hurting herself and her child. Among those few who do develop this disorder, only 4 percent attempt to hurt or kill their children. But the media regularly says wrongly that women with postpartum *depression* may hurt their children, or they mistakenly identify women with postpartum psychosis as having postpartum depression.

In a 2015 story in *Glamour* magazine about actress Hayden Panettiere's postpartum depression, the author writes that Panettiere didn't have the "desire to do harm to the baby, which is one well-known symptom of the condition." This is definitely not a symptom of postpartum depression. The *New York Times* made a similar error in a 2016 news article[11] and the misconstruction is so prevalent that even if you look up the symptoms of postpartum depression on Mayo Clinic's website, they include "thoughts about harming the baby" in their list.[12]

And what is even more confusing and dangerous for the public is the too-common practice of referring to the very few women—with postpartum psychosis—who attempted to, or did indeed, kill their children as having postpartum depression. Throughout a 2014 article in the *Miami Herald* about a woman who tried to kill her two-month-old son, she is referred to as having postpartum depression by the mother, her ob-gyn, and the writer—all saying it was the cause of her homicidal impulses.[13] In 2015, CNN made the same error in a story about postpartum depression that describes three women in New York City who threw their babies out of windows. The article uses that term throughout to describe the mothers' motives, but it's clear they all had a much more serious illness.[14]

## Inflating the Babykiller Problem

Even though such a tiny number of women get postpartum psychosis, and a tiny percentage of those actually harm their children, the media has long covered those stories as if they happen all the time—as if it is a threat all women need to be concerned about. A powerful 1988 *Time* article titled "Why Mothers Kill Their Babies" opened with this introduction: "It is a bizarre and frightening deed, one that elicits an almost primal horror: an apparently normal mother suddenly snaps and kills her newborn child. Sadly, it is not all that rare."[15] No, it is extremely rare! In the same vein, an episode of the television show *Private Practice* aired in 2009 that focused on a woman identified as having postpartum psychosis—at least they got the diagnosis right—who tries to drown her baby. The context the story is told within suggests that all women with this disorder make attempts like this. The truth is that 94 percent of the women who suffer from postpartum psychosis *don't* harm their children, but the salacious, shocking, sensational plotline that they always do is irresistible.

## CASE STORY: THE PORTRAYAL OF ANDREA YATES

The most highly publicized case of a postpartum disorder is Andrea Yates. Her story offers a heartbreaking example of how psychological vulnerability and situational stressors can create the perfect storm of isolation, breakdown, and tragedy. In 2001, as she suffered from postpartum psychosis, Andrea succumbed to voices in her head that told her she threatened the souls of her five children because she had "become Satan himself." To save them from going to hell, she drowned them one by one in the bathtub.

This was an extremely rare event, but the press could not stop writing about it. In a review of articles on "postpartum depression" that appeared from 1998 to 2006 in popular magazines like *Cosmopolitan*, *Good Housekeeping*, *Newsweek*, and *Us Weekly*, researchers found that a third of the articles mention the Andrea Yates case.[16] But, as you will see, what happened to Andrea Yates had nothing to do with postpartum depression—and, most importantly, that the huge majority of women who feel sad after childbirth do not have to worry that they are in danger of harming their children.

By reviewing Andrea's case, I hope to show how a rare disorder like hers develops and reveal just how different it is from postpartum depression. A look at her family and personal histories reveals a textbook case of the internal and external cauldron of postpartum psychosis.[17]

## Personal Psychiatric History

Andrea suffered from postpartum psychosis with hallucinations after the birth of her first child in 1994. She attempted suicide twice in the years between the births of her first and fourth children. After the birth of a fourth child, her care of the children became erratic—she had delusions that they were eating too much and at times refused to feed them. She also had recurrent delusions that there were video cameras in her home and that television characters were communicating with her. She heard voices and began mutilating herself. Some of these episodes brought hospitalization and treatment, but others were not reported to her doctors by Andrea or her husband, Rusty. When she was treated, her care was often inconsistent—even though it is vital that people with such serious symptoms, which remove them from reality, be regularly monitored by psychiatrists.

## Family History

Andrea's father, brother, and sister all have histories of depression, and another brother was diagnosed with bipolar disorder. There is a powerful genetic predisposition, or inclination for, Andrea to suffer from mental illness. A genetic predisposition doesn't guarantee that someone will develop a mental illness, but when you combine it with pressuring social circumstances, the risk that mental illness will develop is much higher. And the pressures on Andrea Yates were intense.

## Situational Stressors

In her marriage, Andrea lived with nonstop stress. Her husband, Rusty, was committed to having as many children as possible and she gave birth to five children in six years. For many years, although they could afford a home, they lived in a Greyhound bus. Andrea's father developed Alzheimer's disease and she was responsible for much of his care. As her children grew older, she homeschooled them. She and Rusty studied with a Christian fundamentalist preacher who emphasized that only repentance could save people from burning in hell, and said that "bad mothers who are going to hell create bad children who will go to hell." These fire and brimstone images may have fueled Andrea's delusion that she was becoming Satan and was hurting her children's souls.

In 2000, she became pregnant with her fifth child. Her psychiatrist was alarmed and warned Andrea and Rusty that her symptoms of postpartum psychosis could be much worse this time. Soon after the baby was born, Andrea's father died and her mental health rapidly deteriorated. She wouldn't feed the baby and stopped talking.

## Repeatedly Unsuccessful Hospitalizations

During the four months that followed, Andrea was hospitalized repeatedly—without much improvement in her symptoms. She rarely spoke, and in group therapy sessions Rusty answered the questions asked of her. The last time she was hospitalized, she was released while still mute, which is an oddity. On July 18, 2001—one month after her release from the hospital—Rusty brought Andrea to see a psychiatrist because her condition was still deteriorating. The doctor adjusted the dosage of her antidepressants, but didn't prescribe any antipsychotics, and told her to "think happy thoughts." Two days later, after Rusty left for work, she methodically drowned all five of her children in the bathtub because she "didn't want her children tormented by Satan" as she was.[18]

This is a tragic story, and I tell it because I want to convey the complex forces at work in the development of this disorder by showing that there were many actions that the people around Andrea could have taken to prevent the deaths of her children. Even with her family and personal psychiatric histories, what happened was by no means inevitable.

## "HOW COULD A MOTHER DO THIS?"

The media coverage and commentary on the Andrea Yates case reflects the simultaneous horror and fascination we feel toward what she did, gives very powerful opinions on why she did it, and argues at length about how she should be dealt with. This case is a community forum onto which people can project their deeply felt values about women and motherhood.

The sheer number of media stories published about this case is remarkable. In the first four weeks after Andrea killed her children, 1,150 articles were published on the event nationally. You may think that it makes sense for such a shocking act to receive that much coverage. But here is an interesting comparison: one year later, a California man who had suffered a long depression killed his five children. In the four weeks afterward, only seventy-seven articles on the story were published nationally.[19] A woman's actions were much more shocking, more a violation of the female, mothering role than his was of the male, fathering role—and this meant it was more worthy of attention.

The articles' descriptions and perspectives on the Andrea Yates case ran with two distinct points of view, which reflect and reveal the polarized discussion in Western culture.

### Feminists Argued That There Was a Deeper Cause

In the liberal and feminist perspective, which portrayed Andrea sympathetically, she is an example of how the model of the all-providing and uncomplaining wife is an unreasonable way to live that can push women to extremes. *Newsweek* columnist Anna Quindlen titled her commentary "Playing God On No Sleep," conveying that this case is a horrifying example of the unreasonable burden that the cult of motherhood brings. The title criticizes the idea that a mother, by herself, should be responsible for the physical and emotional work of parenting, providing whatever her children need by referring to an oft-quoted bromide: "God could not be everywhere, so he made mothers." Her response to this, which she said echoes the thoughts of many other women, was:

> I'm not making excuses for Andrea Yates. I love my children more than life itself. But just because you love people doesn't mean that taking care of them day in and day out isn't often hard, and sometimes even horrible. If God made mothers because he couldn't be everywhere, maybe he could have met us halfway and eradicated vomiting, and colic too, and the hideous sugar-coating of what we are and what we do that leads to false cheer, easy lies and maybe sometimes something much, much worse, almost unimaginable. But not quite.[20]

Groups like the National Organization for Women (NOW) and the ACLU echoed Quindlen's sentiment that the Andrea Yates case brought attention to the patriarchal climate that had created the plight of the suburban housewife. They went on to argue that this societal foundation is also responsible for the dearth of research and resources devoted to postpartum mood disorders. Some mainstream television news shows, like *Today*, took a sympathetic view. When Katie Couric covered the story, she presented Andrea Yates as a victim needing help and offered the phone number for her defense fund in case viewers wished to donate.[21]

## Conservatives Wanted to Throw the Book

The contrasting view presented in the press is that Andrea deserves no sympathy—she was guilty of the murder of her children and needed to be punished. This opinion was espoused by conservatives appalled at the thought that somehow she could be absolved from her crime because mothering is too hard. The managing editor of the *National Review* decried this sympathetic view, writing, "No one is crying out for retribution on behalf of those kids. Give her the chair." When Yates was found not guilty by reason of insanity, a blogger wrote on the website *Independent Conservative*:

> I do not feel that someone should be allowed to get off easy after murdering five babies/children. The fact that she killed five babies/children should be the paramount issue, not deliberating over her mental state. I think she should have been given the

death penalty swiftly after committing the crime and it would discourage others from doing such acts. I also think it would encourage anyone who felt they had a mental issue to seek treatment, before they do something that might result in them getting a death sentence.[22]

The writer presumes that someone having a psychotic break can make rational decisions based on potential consequences like the death penalty. Nothing could be further from the truth. A psychotic break is a departure from reality and reason. Andrea Yates acted on the delusions and hallucinations going on in her mind, not with the rational estimation that she could "get off easy."

A contributor to the conservative women's website *Rightgrrl!* was incensed by the idea that Yates was in any way like other mothers, or that mothering responsibilities could inspire such extremes. Responding to Anna Quindlen's column, Shannon May wrote:

> Motherhood demands extreme sacrifices. They might be quiet sacrifices that continue for years, such as undertaking the nurturing, education, and discipline of one's children instead of pursuing career goals. A mother may need to keep a long, painful vigil as she loves and comforts and protects her dying child. She may be called upon to lay down her life to save her children. While certainly difficult, these things are not inconveniences or nuisances but reasonable and just demands. I pray that a jury will not lose sight of the fact that the five Yates children, who had rightfully expected these things from their mother, instead lost their lives to her selfishness.[23]

The conservative explanation for Andrea's actions—that she was selfish and a criminal, and the liberal feminist explanation—that she was pushed too far by the isolation and burden of caring for five children, both miss the most important reason why she did this. She had postpartum psychosis. She had a severe mental illness. She had voices in her head telling her she was Satan incarnate. Did her circumstances play a role? Yes, but most women who are overwhelmed by circumstances don't kill their children. Is it possible that she was selfish and reasoned that her life would be better without her children? People in a psychotic state don't reason.

# AN ENTRENCHED CONFUSION AT PLAY

The political agendas that played out in the media put Andrea Yates's postpartum psychosis into the background. Instead, the discussion put forth theories of her crime that fit the templates of various ideologies. By doing so, everyone excused themselves from having to get it right. Most articles about this case, liberal and conservative, say she had postpartum depression—not the psychosis she actually had. Rather than educating the public on the rare nature of this disorder and showing how to differentiate it, they chose to politicize and sensationalize a tragic story. Even a decade later, in a story *The Atlantic* published in 2012 that described how Yates was living her life ten years after the death of her children, everyone interviewed and the author himself repeatedly refer to her postpartum depression, not psychosis.[24]

The public's understanding of these disorders is compromised when press coverage gets them consistently wrong. Who gets hurt when postpartum depression is misunderstood, feared, and stigmatized? Everybody. With postpartum depression and postpartum psychosis mixed up in the public consciousness, women who suspect they might have "the illness that makes women kill their children" can be too frightened to admit they are having symptoms and consequently don't get help. Postpartum mood disorders have long-lasting effects on women's mental and physical health, marital quality, adequacy of parenting, and the emotional, social, and cognitive development of their children. If people mistakenly attribute postpartum depression to hormones, they may think it is inevitable and doesn't require treatment. Or they may think that medication is all that is required, rather than providing the tangible and practical help that so many new mothers need. This is another stage in the reproductive life of women where myth is so much louder than fact that we can't even begin to address the real problems.

# CHAPTER 7

# That's Not Me Crying, It Must Be the Baby

When I had my first child, I was waylaid by an unexpected cesarean delivery after many hours of labor, and felt physically and emotionally traumatized. I was unable to feel any happiness about my beautiful, healthy baby girl. When my husband's grandmother came to the hospital to visit, I tried to tell her about the difficult birth, but she cut me off immediately and said, "You have a healthy baby! That's all that matters." I felt as if I just got hit by a car, but nobody noticed the crash. The inability to feel happiness followed me home and was fueled by the terror of not knowing how to take care of a newborn. My mother held the baby and talked to her, and couldn't understand why I didn't do so more. I was so ashamed that I didn't feel the way I was supposed to. In my most private thoughts, I just wanted to run away—which made me feel even more guilty. I met other new mothers but didn't want to tell anyone how sad I was, for fear of being judged. It took me months before I sought professional help. If I had felt more comfortable admitting what I was going through, I'm sure I would have gotten help sooner.

A powerful reason why women hesitate to ask for help with postpartum mood disorders is the fear of failing to live up to the motherhood mystique: the widely held belief that motherhood is "natural, easy, and always enjoyable."[1] The idea that, in addition to being good at caring for children, a woman should enjoy every second of it is a value that is held across cultures. In a comprehensive review, psychologists examined interviews of women with postpartum depression from a wide range of ethnicities and socioeconomic statuses. These interviews included women from diverse countries such as England, Japan, China, India, Uganda, and the

United States. Across the board, these women were ashamed and thought their feelings of despair and loneliness were "unspeakable." Many made a great effort to hide their tears and sadness, which isolated them even further. They found it impossible to share their feelings or ask for help because they thought they had failed to measure up to the ideal of a good mother. The Chinese standard of fulfilling the role of mother with dignity and grace was equally as crushing as the African-American expectation of being strong and capable.[2]

The debilitating emotional symptoms of depression are difficult to bear in any circumstances—with sadness, hopelessness, despair, inability to experience pleasure, and tearfulness—but postpartum depression creates a contradiction that many can't understand or reconcile. Because they have a new baby, mothers are supposed to be extremely happy. Friends and relatives may not permit them to express any of their sadness.

## GETTING THE POSTPARTUM STORY STRAIGHT

So far in this book I've debunked the myths that reproductive events like menstruation and pregnancy cause emotions and behavior that are out of the norm. But many studies indicate that there is indeed increased risk of mood disorders after childbirth.[3] Postpartum depression is a very real phenomenon. And if you read about it in pregnancy guides, women's health websites, and magazine articles, you will be told that—surprise!— hormones are the cause.

They presume that the rapid decline of reproductive hormones, like estrogen and progesterone, are to blame. This seems logical and fits into our view of women's emotions as physically based. However, the research to support this presumption simply isn't there. Thorough reviews of the studies on this done in the last twenty years fail to show a clear link between changes in reproductive hormones and the occurrence of postpartum depression. While it appears that the mental health of a small minority of women is threatened by hormonal change, this is not the case for the great majority of women. In fact, most studies find hormone changes have no role in developing postpartum depression when it does occur.[4]

It's not our hormones after all. But mood changes do happen, and what is most important to debunk here is the stigma that keeps women from seeking help. This chapter is mostly devoted to clarifying the different postpartum experiences and discussing the consequences of women living under the spell of our societal hormone myth.

I mentioned the three types of postpartum mood disorders in the last chapter: postpartum blues, postpartum depression, and postpartum psychosis. I want to discuss each of them more in depth because it is so very important to understand the differences, since their diverse symptoms and causes require different treatments. I also want to help more people learn to distinguish the commonly experienced symptoms from the extreme and dangerous ones so that we do not all fear the worst.

## POSTPARTUM BLUES

When I visited my friend, Bernadette, right after she came home with her new baby, I found her in a puddle of tears in the kitchen. I asked her what was wrong and she said tragically, "I have to make the soup and the can opener is broken. I have to make the soup!" After handling this technological mishap, she calmed down quickly and was back to her normal self. Bernadette was experiencing postpartum blues, a fleeting phenomenon that occurs within the initial ten days after the baby is born. A woman may feel any of the following symptoms at any time in this period: mood swings, tearfulness, irritability, anxiety, and insomnia.[5]

Postpartum blues is very common: psychologists estimate that anywhere from 26 to 85 percent of all new mothers experience it.[6] The cause is unclear. For many years it was assumed that rapidly declining hormone levels were responsible, but research on this question has produced contradictory findings.[7] We do know that having a history of depression before pregnancy and being depressed during pregnancy are risk factors.[8] Fortunately, postpartum blues goes away on its own by the end of the ten days and requires no treatment beyond compassion and some tender, loving care.

## POSTPARTUM DEPRESSION

A more serious mood disorder is postpartum depression. This is a psychological disorder that starts within thirty days of childbirth and lasts for at least two weeks. Sufferers experience the same symptoms the DSM-5 identifies in a major depressive episode that isn't related to childbirth: feeling sad, tearful, hopeless, despairing, having trouble sleeping, suffering from fatigue, and sometimes thinking of suicide.[9] Feelings of anxiety also commonly appear alongside the depressive symptoms. The symptoms can feel overwhelming, making it difficult to function. A woman may have trouble taking care of herself, her baby, and her family. Actress Gwyneth Paltrow vividly described the experience:

> When my son, Moses, came into the world in 2006, I expected to have another period of euphoria following his birth much the way I had when my daughter was born two years earlier. Instead I was confronted with one of the darkest and most painfully debilitating chapters of my life.[10]

Researchers estimate that between 7 and 12 percent of women experience a major depressive episode after childbirth, with an additional 10 percent suffering from mild depression that involves the same symptoms but at a less severe intensity.[11]

The causes for this are well-documented predictors that have psychological, social, and cultural natures.[12] By far the most powerful predictor of postpartum depression is being depressed during pregnancy. This alone accounts for about 40 percent of all cases.[13] So if depression is a problem in a woman's life, having a baby is unlikely to change that because any previous history of depression before becoming pregnant is another risk factor. Experiencing postpartum blues in the first week after the baby is born creates an increased risk for postpartum depression, but it's good to keep in mind that the majority of women who have postpartum blues don't go on to develop postpartum depression.

Social and environmental factors that predict postpartum depression include: stressful life events, childcare stress, poor marital relationship, and poor social support.[14]

## Stressful Life Events

Imagine a new mother who is just keeping her head above water. Despite the sleep deprivation, and amidst mountains of laundry and dirty bottles, she is holding her own and the baby is thriving. But then something else happens that requires more of her emotional or physical attention. She breaks her ankle, her mother gets cancer, her husband loses his job, or her older child gets suspended from school. Stressful life events threaten the mental health of people who *didn't* just have a baby because they are not under our control. So they can push a woman's already-taxed emotional resources beyond the brink.

## Childcare Stress

New babies are fragile. They barely seem able to exist without attention to their every need and can only communicate those needs by crying. All the new things mothers need to do to provide that care, like feeding, diapering, cleaning, and soothing, may or may not happen easily. Learning how to breastfeed is not the straightforward skill it appears to be: there are babies who won't latch on, and women get sore nipples or infected milk ducts. Expand that to a baby who is colicky, rarely naps, or will not sleep for more than two hours at a time—all of these lead to a deliriously sleep-deprived mother. When these kinds of stressors pile up, vulnerability to depression increases.

## Poor Marital Relationship

Women can be dealing with all of these new and unpredictable responsibilities in the context of a troubled marriage. I cringe when I hear stories of couples who decided to have a baby to save their marriage. If a relationship has tension, fighting, distrust, and a lack of cooperation, bringing a new baby into it is like pouring gasoline on a fire. Even solid marriages are strained by the needs of caring for a newborn baby. When women don't have a solid relationship to rely on, it may not withstand the stresses a new baby brings. A woman in this situation may fear for the future and, especially if she relies on the father financially, worry about how she would manage if her marriage were to crumble irreparably.

## Poor Social Support

It's not unusual for Americans to move far from where they grew up and to lose the support that nearby family can provide. There is nothing like the stress-free confidence of leaving a child with grandparents. When my first daughter was three weeks old, my mother said to me, "You look tired; I'm taking that baby tonight." What a godsend! Grandparents can be absolutely devoted to a new baby, and their help offers huge respite from the round-the-clock job of motherhood. If a friend can come over for an hour just so a new mother can shower, or someone makes a point to ask how she's doing, it can make a big difference. When women don't have people in their lives who can provide that kind of respite, the never-ending responsibility of newborn care can overwhelm them. A social circle, or lack of one, has a strong influence on the ability to cope.

This list of predictors might make you question why a scientist needs to verify the obvious—who wouldn't feel some depression? The experience of it could even be a signal that a woman needs to devote more energy toward caring for herself in the midst of her new role. But that would go against our cultural notions of a good mother. These social variables are well-established contributors. The fact that they are all subject to change, to some degree, says that the number of women who suffer from postpartum depression can be reduced by altering them.

Culturally, psychologists have found that women are more likely to develop postpartum depression when they live in areas where there is a lack of birth control availability and they are forced to have unwanted pregnancies. If it is considered immoral or illegal for women to control when and how often they become pregnant, some women will have pregnancies they don't want. And if there is a widespread preference for a male child, like in Southeast Asia, and a girl is born, a woman may feel disappointed—even in herself. For these cultures, there is a higher risk of postpartum depression when women give birth to girls.[15] Cultures create the boundaries we live in and assign meaning to actions and events—creating the potential for happiness or distress. Everything humans do, we do in a cultural context.

Fortunately, a variety of treatment options successfully bring women relief from postpartum depression. Many different types of psychotherapy have proven effective on an individual basis, or with the participation of her partner or spouse. Antidepressant medication is also highly effective in treating these symptoms, and success rates improve when antidepressants and psychotherapy are combined. For women who are breastfeeding, however, taking antidepressants may be problematic because the medication is passed along to the infant through breast milk. The degree to which this medication can harm the infant is unknown because there are no randomized studies examining this question,[16] as it would be unethical to randomly assign a woman to take medication that might threaten the health of her child. So physicians and their patients must carefully navigate the potential risks and benefits of all treatment options.

As common sense would dictate, depressed mothers also do better when they are given help from friends and family to ease the strains of caring for a newborn and recovering from childbirth. Participation in support groups also provides emotional support and understanding, as well as tangible support with solutions to the universal challenges women face during this time.

## POSTPARTUM PSYCHOSIS

As I made clear in chapter 6, postpartum psychosis is an extremely rare disorder that affects one in one-thousand women. It strikes within the first thirty days after childbirth and the symptoms are severe, come on suddenly, and involve a psychotic break with reality. A woman may experience hallucinations and delusions, and have extreme and unpredictable mood swings from manic elation to deadening sadness. She may hear voices, be confused, and have thoughts of harming herself or her child.[17]

It is imperative that a woman diagnosed with postpartum psychosis be immediately hospitalized to stabilize her condition. She is likely to be prescribed antipsychotic medication like Risperdal to stop her delusions and hallucinations, a mood stabilizer like Lithium, or tranquilizers like Valium to calm her agitation. If the mother is breastfeeding, the potential risks and benefits of each drug must be weighed. In such an extreme situation, however, maintaining breastfeeding may be seen as a secondary consideration to stabilizing a mother's mental health. The prognosis for women with postpartum psychosis is commonly positive, but the risk for a recurrence with future pregnancies is high.[18]

It is difficult to know what causes a woman to develop postpartum psychosis because so few women have this condition, making it impossible to do systematic, randomized studies. At the same time, examining medical records and interviewing women who have had postpartum psychosis has revealed some consistent risk factors. Postpartum psychosis is likely to develop as the result of a combination of factors that create a dangerous storm of mental illness—often a strong, genetic predisposition that interacts with the physical and emotional stress of childbirth. The most well-documented risk factors are:[19]

- Being diagnosed with bipolar disorder prior to delivery

- Being diagnosed with bipolar disorder and having had a previous episode of postpartum psychosis, or a family history of postpartum psychosis

- Having family members who have mood disorders or have been hospitalized for psychiatric reasons

- Death of the infant

- Perceived lack of support from partner

- Marital conflict

Bipolar disorder used to be called "manic depression," and it is a chronic mood disorder in which periods of intense elation and energy alternate with periods of intense sadness and hopelessness. Without medication, daily functioning can be severely compromised.[20] Women with previously diagnosed bipolar disorder have a one-in-four chance of developing postpartum psychosis. Of those women, if they suffered from psychosis after a previous pregnancy or have a family member who has, there is a one-in-two chance that they will experience a psychotic break after childbirth.

As you can imagine, a death of the baby soon after delivery is psychologically devastating and increases the risk of postpartum psychosis. And it is clear that situational stressors, like having marital difficulties and feeling unsupported in caring for the child, play a role as well.

With these discussions, I hope you can see how damaging the hormone myth is in postpartum. It affirms the idea that any kind of postpartum mood disorder is because of biology—hormones, of course—and that a woman should try to just shake it off. The reality is way more complicated than that. A woman's psychological history and the situation she lives in, the quality of her marriage and the extent of support she gets, are much more important factors that cause postpartum mood disorders than hormones. The idea that good women always love being mothers brings us to the unavoidable conclusion that we must be bad women for feeling anything else, which keeps us from seeking help. And not getting help hurts everyone.

# CONSEQUENCES OF NOT SEEKING TREATMENT

Postpartum blues is transient and goes away on its own without any treatment, but postpartum depression and postpartum psychosis can have long-lasting consequences, especially if left untreated. While the repercussions of untreated postpartum depression are far-reaching, the consequences of untreated postpartum psychosis can be catastrophic. Thankfully, postpartum psychosis is extremely rare, and with the early treatment of hospitalization, antipsychotic drugs, and strong social support, the prognosis is commonly positive.[21] However, without treatment, the risks to the mother and her child escalate.

## Risks to the Mother

Depression is no picnic. As you can imagine, postpartum depression has wide-ranging effects on a new mother. Physically, it increases her risk of cardiovascular disease: a woman with postpartum depression, who has no previous history of heart disease, has four-and-a-half times the risk of having a heart attack compared to women who are not depressed. Depression compromises the immune system by decreasing the production of white blood cells. Also, feeling hopeless and full of self-loathing doesn't lead to making healthy choices—she is more likely to abuse alcohol and drugs, use tobacco, and have poor nutrition, and less likely to participate in preventive health behaviors like using seat belts or sunscreen.[22] As any mother knows, adding a baby to the family is challenging under the best circumstances with nonstop care for a newborn, household chores, attending to other children, and perhaps going back to work after a brief maternity leave. Doing so under the heavy weight of depression would deplete anyone's emotional and physical resources.

Women suffering from postpartum psychosis experience all of this, plus a psychotic break with reality, and it's common to think about suicide.

For her, the risk of suicide in the year after she gives birth is substantially higher than the general female population.[23] After interviewing women who had had postpartum psychosis, one researcher described the hopelessness they felt:

> The women stated that they felt as if all the doors were closed and they had entered total darkness where no improvement could be seen. They felt they were beyond rescue...and without any hope... Only one thing saved them from suicide and that was the thought of leaving their families behind to mourn.[24]

It's clear from the interviews that these women weren't beyond help or hope, and with appropriate treatment and the support of loving family members, they were able to heal and return to normal functioning. But to get to treatment, they and their loved ones had to get past the stigma and shame generally attached to having challenges postpartum.

## Risks to Children

It's no coincidence that most parents want to gaze into a baby's eyes and naturally respond to them. What feels like a natural, loving interaction forms the foundation for emotional and mental health. A depressed mother tends to interact with her baby differently, which can have long-term developmental ramifications. She spends less time in prolonged eye contact with the baby, is less responsive to the baby's initiations of contact through gurgling, babbling, or crying, and shows more negative and less positive facial expressions to the baby.[25]

The ways that depressed mothers interact—or fail to interact—with their babies have direct effects on emotional, cognitive, and social development. Infants of depressed mothers are slower to develop a secure attachment to the mother, as well as appropriate emotional expression and management. They are more reactive to stress, more fussy, less playful,[26] have lower scores in motor development, are less content, and are perceived by their mothers as more difficult to care for compared to the children of nondepressed mothers.[27] The developmental deficiencies, when compared to children with mothers who did not experience depression, don't stop in infancy. Preschoolers score lower on intelligence tests and have more behavioral problems.[28] School-age children are more likely to show depressive symptoms, have smaller vocabularies, and lower social competence. By age thirteen, these children also have lower IQ scores and are more likely to be in special education classes.[29]

When a woman suffers from postpartum depression, not only does her infant suffer, but any older siblings are at risk as well. Children are sensitive beings: they notice when a previously fun and affectionate mother becomes remote and moody. Depression disrupts a woman's ability to be an attentive, affectionate parent, so when depression persists, the mental health of all her children is compromised. Older children of depressed mothers have higher rates of anxiety and behavioral problems, more negative moods, are more vulnerable to developing depression, score lower on IQ tests, have lower overall academic performance, and are more likely to be excluded by peers.[30] Overall, children of mothers who had postpartum depression are at a higher risk of behavioral problems, deficient social skills, cognitive difficulties, and later psychological disorders—throughout their childhood and beyond.[31]

A woman with postpartum psychosis may experience such severe depression that she can't get out of bed. She may have delusions or hallucinations that make her more likely to neglect or abuse her baby. She may imagine that she fed him an hour ago, when it was in fact five hours ago. She may stay away from her baby because she hears voices telling her she is a bad mother and can only hurt her baby.[32] It's not uncommon for a woman with postpartum psychosis to have *thoughts* of killing her child, although only 4 percent of these women actually do so.[33] I know any sentence with the phrase "thoughts of killing her child" is terrifying to read, but 96 percent of women with postpartum psychosis *don't* kill their children. This is a small risk, but obviously has to be taken seriously.

## Risks to Relationships

The birth of a child, particularly a first child, is a time of stress for many couples. For a variety of reasons, the majority of couples suffer a decline in relationship satisfaction when a child is born. When my first daughter was born, I wanted to hang onto my husband's leg as he left to go to work, and I wanted to cry out: "Don't leave me alone to care for this baby!" I was a graduate student and it made sense for me to take off a semester when she was born. But I was so jealous that he got to leave every day. Yes, he was going to work so we could pay our mortgage and have food, but the combination of my complete ignorance of how to take care of a baby and her unsoothable colic made each day feel like being left alone to walk through a minefield. Was she hungry? Did she need her diaper changed? Was gas bothering her? The answers never seemed clear. I felt like I was failing daily and was angry that he didn't have to go through this with me. And believe me, when he came home, he did plenty! He took the baby, fed her, changed diapers—the whole nine yards. But he got to escape for eight hours a day, which made me resentful and fairly unpleasant to be with.

These feelings are exacerbated if one parent is doing less than the other parent expects. The grueling physical work of infant care, the lack of sleep, and the upending of expectations can all contribute to new parents' frustration and resentment.[34] Adding postpartum depression to the mix puts inevitable pressures on the relationship. Depression, anxiety, sleep deprivation, and resentment are a toxic brew.

Even without the birth of a child, one partner's depression is strongly related to decreased quality of relationship and higher rates of divorce.[35] Some of this can be explained by the particular behaviors of depressed people and the behaviors they elicit from others. My husband and I were heading down this road. When he suggested that napping when the baby slept might make me feel better, I said, "Oh really?! When am I supposed to shower or do the dishes or deal with the piles of clothes caked in spit up?" I thought he was being critical and he thought I was jumping down his throat. In general, the interactions of couples when one is depressed are more negative, and those who are depressed can be highly reactive to criticism.[36] Their complaints of physical and psychological distress, and their displays of sadness, can provoke behavior from their partner that produces more stress. Those in relationships with depressed people are more likely to see them as a burden, and to reject and criticize them, producing more—rather than less—conflict.[37]

Luckily, treatment for depression is very effective. Whether it's therapy with a trained psychologist or antidepressants prescribed by a physician or psychiatrist, treating depression is something that these professionals have had success at and for which they have a lot of tools at their disposal.[38] But to get treatment and avoid many of these potential negative consequences, people need to understand what postpartum depression is—and not fear admitting they have it.

The foundation of the hormone myth here—that women are biologically made to be nurturing, happy mothers—makes it especially difficult for women to admit they are depressed. Who wants to feel like she is being a bad, unnatural mother? The fear of being honest about how hard mothering is keeps women from admitting they are hurting, and exposes them and their families to dangerous and long-lasting risks.

## THE EFFECTS OF RESOURCES AND SUPPORT

This fear is something that is in everyone's power to change. We can change our views. Rather than thinking of the arrival of a new baby as a private situation, we can think of new mothers as in need of community resources. In colonial times, when a woman had a baby, neighbors and friends took turns feeding her family and doing her chores so she could properly recover and bond with her baby. We can do that for each other. Merely saying "Call me if you need help" doesn't help, because American individualism makes us resist presenting ourselves as needy. It's better to say, "I'm going to come over on Tuesday and Thursday this week to bring dinner—what is a good time to drop it off?" This makes it a fait accompli and the new mother only has to say what time is best.

Women with newborn babies need sympathy and understanding for this phenomenal responsibility they now have—and concrete help. If many people in her world pitched in, her mental health would benefit and she would be less vulnerable to developing postpartum depression.

## IF WE ALL GOT REAL ABOUT MOTHERHOOD

Part and parcel of this approach is having a realistic perspective on mothering. It means leaving the biological imperatives of the hormone myth behind and rejecting the idea that women are biologically made to be selfless, mothering machines who have a natural instinct for knowing how to mother and a natural impulse to love every minute of it. Caring for a newborn is hard, and involves a skillset that, these days, most don't learn beforehand. Women need to feel comfortable asking for, and receiving, help without feeling like a bad mother. Let's stop blaming these struggles on hormones and start making new mothers' lives more reasonable by expecting more from husbands and everyone in their social circle.

I know that when I finally asked for help from friends and family, and I was able to feel like I wasn't in it alone, my postpartum depression eased. It is in our power to improve new mothers' mental health and, therefore, the health of their children. It only requires our rejection of the hormone myth and an embrace of our communal commitment to supporting women during what is, in reality, a difficult time of life.

# CHAPTER 8

# The Reputation of Menopause Precedes It

Television has been in the forefront of presenting menopause as the end of femininity and our very identities as women. In 1972, an *All in the Family* episode called "Edith's Problem" was seen as groundbreaking for addressing the topic of menopause. When Edith finds out she is going through "the change," and her daughter, Gloria, suggests that it is a "natural, beautiful time of life," Edith says: "Beautiful? Well I don't feel very beautiful… When Archie hears about this he ain't gonna love me no more."[1] The image hasn't changed much: in 2000, when Samantha of *Sex and the City* suspects she is entering menopause because her period is late, she says, "I'm day-old bread and my time is up."

Menopause. The very word conjures images of wrinkled and undesirable women who are way past their prime. It is a cultural mark of getting old, which is a fate we must run from. We cannot look at a magazine or website or Facebook ad without getting bombarded with the message that we must try to appear younger than we are—and of course buy the products and services that will help us do so. Our response is pretty crazy because whatever we do, we can't stop time. But we live in a youth-oriented culture. Particularly for women, being young means being beautiful, exciting, active, and relevant. Being old is to be boring, uninvolved, wrinkled and therefore ugly, and ultimately irrelevant.[2]

To maintain self-esteem as we age is challenging. I will admit that I can't help but be pleased when people are amazed that I'm in my fifties. I dye my grey hair back to brown, use age-defying face cream, and put a huge amount of effort into staying trim, if not thin. And the irony is that

I like the age I'm at. So far, my fifties have been everything I've hoped for: a time of passionate work productivity and devotion to my personal interests and needs. I know who I am and what I want, and—more importantly—what I don't want. But I still can't escape the desire to appear younger. And nothing heralds getting older like the beginning of menopause. It is an unavoidable progression of events that happen as we enter midlife.

The social meaning of menopause in Western nations is one of decay and illness. It marks a time when women are thought to lose desirability and must leave the game of attraction and sex behind—all of which can affect our identities as women.[3] The television characters I quoted aren't addressing the physical symptoms of menopause; instead, they speak to the plummeting value of older women. In a simultaneously tragic and hilarious television skit, Amy Schumer scathingly depicts this fate when she runs into middle-aged actresses Tina Fey, Julia Louis-Dreyfus, and Patricia Arquette—arguably three very attractive women. To Amy's horror, they are celebrating Julia's "last fuckable day"—the day the media arbitrarily decides that an actress is no longer believably desirable.[4] Schumer is skewering the reality of cultural ideals, in which women of menopausal age get demoted to sexless crones.

## MENOPAUSE IS A MODERN ILLNESS

These attitudes about menopause are relatively new in human history. The oldest reference to menopause is found in Genesis, when Sarah is described as "past the age of childbearing."[5] In the premodern era when health was understood in terms of the four humors, it was thought that humors harden as a woman ages, causing the end of menstruation.[6] But for most of human history women generally didn't live past forty-five years old, so before the nineteenth and twentieth centuries brought longer life spans, menopause was known but rare.[7]

In the late 1800s, the establishment of the modern medical field in the United States and Europe was taking hold and physicians started wielding cultural authority over health issues. Rather than mothers and midwives modeling and advising women about reproductive health, graduates from newly minted medical schools confidently instructed their patients, and the public, on the proper care of women's bodies.[8] These doctors understood menopause as a milestone in a woman's reproductive life, but regarded it as one that came with no serious health problems. Medical textbooks of the time didn't even cover the topic. Many saw menopause as an opportunity for women to engage in, and contribute to, society outside of the home—in ways that didn't infringe on caring for a husband or threatening his status as breadwinner. By the 1930s and 1940s, menopause began to be discussed in nursing and medical journals, but they reported that most women didn't experience symptoms troubling enough to require medical attention.[9]

## THE NEED FOR FEMININITY MAINTENANCE

It is only recently that people began thinking about menopause as a disease in need of treatment. In the 1950s, the whole discussion took on a much different tone. Doctors warned that menopause brought "emotional turmoil" and could "threaten a family's tranquility," citing examples of menopausal women getting annoyed with their husbands and complaining about doing housework. This was clearly not acceptable, and the popular advice literature told women to get a hold of themselves and control their feelings. If they found that to be impossible, one female physician recommended that they simply pretend they didn't feel that way.[10] The whole discourse evaded any notion that women may be upset for other reasons, valid reasons, and made no effort to figure out why they were dissatisfied.

This is when the thought originated that the onset of menopause causes accelerated aging in the female body and a decline of attractiveness. Medical experts warned that menopausal women get "pouchy stomachs" and "saggy breasts," and that they needed to work hard to maintain their attractiveness because it is "part of the marital bargain."[11]

The marital bargain? If you've ever thought the radical feminist description of marriage as "legalized prostitution" is extreme, well here is the inspiration in living color. The understanding that a man agrees to marry and financially support a woman if she remains attractive and sexually available encapsulates much of the rhetoric about menopause at this time. Rather than considering a woman's physical and emotional health as important aspects of her well-being, the medical community was more concerned about maintaining her femininity during and after menopause to tend to her husband's happiness. And the era believed his happiness was reliant on having a compliant, domestic, attractive, sexual partner.

The myth that menopause made women sick, ugly, and unpleasant was ultimately legitimized and popularized in 1966 when gynecologist Robert A. Wilson's book called *Feminine Forever* was published. I can only describe this book as an unbelievable compendium of misogyny and chauvinism. Throughout, the author emphasized the fundamental importance of women's attractiveness with lines like "A woman's physical appeal is her starting capital in the venture of life—the ante which lets her into the game." Wilson sympathized and damned menopausal women with the comment: "No woman can escape the horror of this living decay," as he declared that the decline of estrogen will inevitably make "breasts become flabby and the vagina becomes stiff and unyielding."

He argued that, psychologically, menopause could push women into two very different—but equally undesirable—states. He recounted many stories of husbands who found their menopausal wives to be crabby, refusing to make dinner. Wilson sympathized, and said that decreased estrogen can make a woman become a "dull-minded, sharp-tongued caricature of her former self." On the other hand, he warned that a menopausal woman can also eventually "subside into an uneasy apathy that is indeed a form of death within life." In this state, he explained that a woman can "acquire a vapid cow-like feeling" in which the "world appears as though through a grey veil, and they live as docile harmless creatures missing most of life's values."[11] Not an attractive picture either way.

## HORMONES TO THE RESCUE

Wilson argued that menopause is a hormone-deficiency disease, and that to save women and their husbands from misery, all women—even those without symptoms—should take synthetic hormones for the remainder of their lives. With hormone replacement therapy, he said that women could avoid "the death of their own womanhood" and stay "feminine forever."

The hormones Wilson wrote about first came to market in the early 1940s, after the pharmaceutical company Ayerst Laboratories developed a cost-effective form, called Premarin, that consists of estrogen extracted from pregnant mares' urine. Premarin was originally prescribed only to treat women who experienced menopausal symptoms, like hot flashes, as disturbing. But after the publication of *Feminine Forever*, with its wide popularity with both readers and the media, Premarin sales doubled from 1960 to 1975, eventually bringing billions of dollars in profit.[13]

Advertisements for Premarin that were released in 1960s medical journals featured glamorous, attractive, middle-aged women being adored by their equally attractive husbands—ostensibly because these ladies stayed youthful and vibrant thanks to hormones. The ads simply scream: "Look what hormones can do!" One Premarin ad ran with the headline "Husbands, too, like Premarin," which went on to deliver the message that men deserve a pleasant and reasonable woman—which Premarin could ensure. Under a picture of a happy and attractive middle-aged couple on a sailboat, the text read:

> The physician who puts a woman on "Premarin" when she is suffering from menopause usually makes her pleasant to live with once again. It is no easy thing for a man to take the stings and barbs of business life, then to come home to the turmoil of a woman "going through the change of life." If she is not on "Premarin," that is.

In the 1970s, the ads emphasized what horrors happen when middle-aged women *don't* take hormones. No longer glamorous and glowing, the menopausal women shown were wrinkled and ugly. One featured a dowdy grandmother bemoaning the fact that her husband, at the height of his career, no longer had time for her. The message was that if she took Premarin, she would be young and attractive again, and her husband would find her worthy of attention.[14] This change in tone was a result of the women's health movement of the 1960s and 1970s, which encouraged women to become more active participants in their healthcare,[15] so women needed to be exhorted to choose to pursue hormone replacement therapy.

The women's health movement was based on the popular premise of "question authority." It resisted the perception of doctors as all-knowing authorities who dictated what was best for women, and promoted the idea that women could and should be informed participants in their health care decisions. This philosophy was best captured in the 1969 publication of *Our Bodies, Ourselves*, a compendium of accessible information about women's health—especially women's reproductive health—that continues to provide multiple perspectives on how to stay healthy and how to treat illnesses particular to women. In 1985, women's health activists successfully lobbied Congress to require anyone doing a clinical health trial with a government grant to include women as study participants. Previous to that, most studies that physicians used to guide their treatment choices for women included only male participants. There were vast gaps of knowledge about women's health because of this bias, and the women's health movement helped to close that gap.[16]

Premarin ads appealed to this popular idea of patients as informed consumers. A commercial in the 1990s featured a doctor saying, "Speak to your doctor about what you can do to protect your health during and after menopause."[17] They were still selling women a drug that could harm their health, as I'll discuss in chapter 10, but now they did it under the guise of encouraging women to take control of menopause. This attitude took root in our culture and the self-help books and popular media throughout the 1980s and 1990s continued to represent menopause as a terrifying illness.[18]

## MYTHIC ATTITUDES ABOUT MENOPAUSE MAKE IT SO

The current best-selling books on Amazon.com about menopause all present it as a stage of life that brings physical and emotional harms that a woman must battle with. Titles like *Before the Change: Taking Charge of Your Perimenopause*, *The Hormone Cure*, and even Mayo Clinic's *The Menopause Solution* position menopause as a threatening illness that needs to be actively dealt with. Very few, like Christiane Northrup's books *The Secret Pleasures of Menopause* and *The Wisdom of Menopause*, consider positive aspects of menopause.

Positive aspects of menopause? Imagine that. In chapter 9, I'll show that they are not only possible, but that they are experiences the vast majority of women actually have. Remember the discussion about how negative attitudes and expectations about menstruation are related to actually having a worse experience? This is also the case with menopause.[19] Premenopausal women who think that menopause makes women less attractive and more likely to need medical treatment report physical symptoms of menopause, like hot flashes and disturbed sleep, more often and more severely than women with positive attitudes. These negative attitudes about menopause also predict feelings of distress and depression during the menopause years.[20] Here are the major social forces that influence a woman's perception of menopause.

## Spousal Responses

Women's attitudes may be influenced by how their partners respond to this transition. In interviews with sixty-one menopausal women, one researcher found it a recurring theme that men were encouraging women to interpret their symptoms as an illness and pressuring them to get the illness fixed.[21] Many men were disturbed by their wives' hot flashes and menstrual changes, and were exasperated by the women's inability to control their bodies. Of course, there are some men who want to be supportive, but unfortunately most men don't have accurate information about the process of menopause and aren't sure how to be helpful.[22]

## Generational Norms

Generational norms may affect how a woman interprets and experiences menopause. A study of white, middle-class baby boomers and their mothers, who were born in the 1920s and 1930s, found that the daughters and mothers had very similar physical symptoms of menopause. But there were fascinating differences in how each group thought about, and experienced, that time of life.[23] The mothers were born in a time when no one spoke publicly about issues like menopause or sexuality. They accepted menopause simply as a stage of life and few sought any medical treatment. Most of the mothers expressed feeling excitement at that time; since reproduction was over, they would have the opportunity to focus on themselves.

Their baby-boomer daughters approached menopause quite differently. They talked about it with anybody and everybody—including their friends, family, coworkers, husbands, and physicians—and some joined support groups to provide a forum for discussion. They feared menopause. They saw it as connected to aging and the end of attractiveness, and felt it was a health problem that needed curing. A common theme was a desire to control their bodies, and they expressed pride in all the ways they had worked to delay, or minimize, the onset of menopause and other physical signs of aging. They used over-the-counter drugs, antiaging products, and almost all of them used hormone replacement therapy—even though it is now highly controversial and can cause the serious, long-term health risks that I discuss in chapter 10.[24] For these women, menopause didn't represent the end of reproduction because they had access to birth control methods throughout their reproductive years, while their mothers did not. The results of this study offer an example of how the same physical symptoms can bring distress or not, based on different sensibilities about aging, expected control of one's health, and openness about reproductive events.

## Racial and Cultural Norms

There are a wide variety of attitudes that women have about menopause, which depend on their background and the culture in which they live. In the United States, African-American women have a more positive attitude toward menopause than European-American women and Latina women, with Asian-American women having the least positive attitudes.[25] Women living in Japan have much more positive attitudes about menopause than women in Western nations, possibly because they report fewer physical symptoms. Women in nations like Greece, Mexico, and India have generally positive views, especially where older women are valued.[26]

## Being Exposed to Positive Views

It appears that women's attitudes about menopause are changeable. One study provided an education program to eighty women between forty and sixty years old. The women met ten times for two hours, and in that time menopause was presented as a natural part of life. Medical professionals presented ways to prevent illness and to promote physical, emotional, and social health. At the end of the ten sessions, participants reported not only more positive attitudes about menopause, but also a decrease in physical and psychological symptoms experienced.[27]

As the authors of the study point out, although there is considerable evidence for the major role of attitudes in predicting a woman's experience of menopause, doctors continue to address patients as though it is a sickness requiring medical treatment, rather than promoting a positive attitude and encouraging a healthy lifestyle. So, for the rest of this chapter I want to step outside the cultural overlays and personal influences and look at what, exactly, happens to a woman's body during this time. Because while there are many psychological, social, and situational factors that dictate how it is experienced physically and emotionally, it is fundamentally a biological process.

## WHAT HAPPENS TO THE BODY DURING THE MENOPAUSAL YEARS

It's important to understand what happens—and what doesn't happen—biologically to see menopause for what it is: a time of natural, biological changes that simply represents a new stage in a woman's reproductive health and generally is not experienced as, or needs to be treated as, an illness. To support this view, I'll share some facts about what happens in a woman's body when she is going through this transition.

Throughout a woman's childbearing years, her reproductive system creates an amazing concert of potential and replenishment. When she reaches middle age, subtle hormonal and physiological changes begin to occur that indicate the beginning of a new stage of life. The word "menopause" has generally been used to refer to several years of reproductive change that brings the end of menstrual periods and the beginning of nonchildbearing years—though the medical community has developed more specific language to refer to the different stages of this transition.[28] The following stage-based terms only refer to a woman who is not taking hormones and has not had a hysterectomy, as those interventions cause changes to the experience.

### Premenopause

A woman is referred to as *premenopausal* when she has had regular periods for at least the last three months, and has had no changes in her regularity. Her hormones levels are maintained at the level that facilitates monthly menstruation. This is when her menstrual cycle is chugging along like it always has and her fertility needs to be managed with birth control.

## Perimenopause, or the Menopause Transition

This is when changes begin that can take place over a period of five to ten years. The average age a woman enters the menopause transition is fifty-one, although the range is forty-five to fifty-five.[29] A woman's period starts to skip around irregularly. Researchers define *early transition* as when a woman starts to see changes in the length of her period for at least two cycles in the last year. Her ovaries produce fewer follicles and estrogen levels begin to fluctuate. *Late transition* is marked by more irregular periods, a heavy flow, and at least three missed periods in the last year. Estrogen levels decline, and follicle-stimulating hormone (FSH) and luteinizing hormone (LH) increase. Ovulation, though less frequent, can still occur.

## Postmenopause

A woman is said to be postmenopausal when she has had no menstrual periods for the last twelve months. Estrogen produced by the ovaries continues to decline, but it is still produced in muscle and fat tissue. Only at this point can a woman confidently stop using birth control.

## PHYSICAL EXPERIENCES A WOMAN MAY, OR MAY NOT, HAVE

There is a wide variety of ways women physically experience the menopause transition stage. Some have no symptoms and some have many.[30] For those who do experience symptoms, the most common for American women are hot flashes, vaginal dryness, sleep problems, and headaches.[31] Women who take hormone replacement therapy have substantially fewer hot flashes and vaginal dryness than women who do not.[32] Women who have radical hysterectomies, which remove their ovaries and uterus, experience more sudden and severe physical symptoms of menopause than those who begin menopause naturally.[33]

About 25 percent of North American and European women describe their symptoms as sometimes severe.[34] Overall, Japanese women report much fewer symptoms at menopause compared to North American women,[35] but studies find that Japanese women who live in urban areas experience hot flashes at the same rate as North American women and

Japanese women living in rural areas experience them at a much lower rate.[36] Perhaps a more Westernized lifestyle contributes to hot flashes. In India, the most common symptoms are fatigue and achiness in muscles and joints.[37] For a phenomenon that is biological, a wide range of factors do influence who will experience symptoms and how severely. Race, ethnicity, education level, health behaviors, stress level, and depression all play a role. American Hispanic women report headaches the most, with Asian-Americans reporting the least. Hot flashes are reported by African-American women the most and Asian-American women the least.[38]

I want to spend some time discussing the most common physical symptoms women experience and the biggest health risks that develop during the menopausal years, to give you a sense of how changing hormones affect women, on a basic level, and also how easy it can be to manage these changes with minimally invasive adjustments.

## Hot Flashes

The most commonly experienced physical symptom during the menopausal transition and postmenopause is the hot flash. Hot flashes happen when blood vessels close to the skin dilate. They involve a sudden feeling of increased internal warmth that rises through the body and often results in sweating and flushed skin. It appears that hot flashes are caused by declining estrogen, but it is probably more complicated than that because the estrogen of every woman who goes through the menopause transition declines, but not every woman gets hot flashes.[39] They can persist for several years, and their intensity ranges from minor to feeling as if on fire. When I started getting hot flashes, I was on an airplane and felt very confused. I'm always cold when I fly, but not this time. I said to my daughter "Oh my God! How did it get so hot in here?" I was sweating profusely from head to toe. My daughter turned to me and gently said, "It's not hot in here Ma, it's you." And there it was. I have since learned to dress in layers and to take comfort in knowing that, yes, my hot flashes are hot—but they do pass.

## Disrupted Sleep

Another common symptom reported during the menopausal transition is disturbed sleep. This is mostly because of hot flashes at night, better known as "night sweats."[40] It can be annoying for the many women who wake up covered in sweat several times a night and get out of bed in the morning feeling as if they didn't sleep at all. There are a variety of ways to decrease night sweats, such as keeping the bedroom at a cool temperature and sleeping in light, cotton pajamas. Exercising just thirty minutes a day can also help decrease the number of hot flashes women experience.[41]

## Headaches

Just as hot flashes play a role in insomnia, insomnia can play a role in menopausal migraine headaches. A migraine is a debilitating headache that lasts anywhere from four hours to two days. Along with the pain, migraine sufferers can experience intense sensitivity to light and noise, with nausea and vomiting.[42] At any time of life, insomnia can be a trigger for a migraine, so women with disrupted sleep because of night sweats are equally at risk.[43] Other women at risk for migraines during the menopause transition are those who had a surgical, rather than natural, menopause and those who had migraines related to their menstrual cycle premenopausally. The frequency of migraines is highest during the late menopausal transition, but postmenopause brings a substantial reduction of headaches to below the premenopausal level.[44] Neurologists find that even though these headaches are related to changes in estrogen, estrogen replacement therapy is not an effective treatment and can worsen symptoms, therefore, nonhormonal migraine treatments are optimal.[45]

## Vaginal Dryness

The decline in estrogen causes some women to experience vaginal drying. The vaginal tissue becomes thinner and there is less natural lubrication, sometimes causing painful intercourse.[46] There are many lubricants sold over the counter that can address this problem, although some women do feel the need to seek medical treatment and find relief with a limited course of hormonal cream. Alternately, some women find this to be a time when they develop new ways to be intimate or experience sexual satisfaction.[47] Oral sex and other kinds of stimulation bring women immense pleasure, and sensual massage can be a way to have intimate physical and emotional contact.

## Heart Disease

Women's risk for developing cardiovascular disease substantially increases after menopause begins and is the leading cause of death, as 22 percent of women will die from it. Ten years after the beginning of the menopause transition, the risk for having a heart attack *quadruples*.[48] Two major reasons why menopause increases the risk of heart disease are changes in body fat and changes in cholesterol levels.[49] In the menopausal years, the fat in women's bodies gets redistributed from mainly in their lower bodies to their upper bodies, changing from pear-shaped to apple-shaped. Carrying fat in the upper body has been long known to be a risk factor for heart disease.[50] Also, the decrease in estrogen levels cause women's "bad" cholesterol (LDL) to go up and "good" cholesterol (HDL) to go down, increasing their risk for heart disease. The good news is that it is not inevitable for anyone to develop heart disease. Lifestyle choices have a substantial impact on risk and physicians confidently know that maintaining a healthy weight and diet, regular exercise, and refraining from smoking powerfully reduce a person's risk of developing heart disease, whether they are postmenopausal or not.[51]

## Breast Cancer

When looking at the big picture of women's health, it's important to keep in mind that breast cancer causes only 3 *percent* of the total annual deaths of American women.[52] Despite this fact, only about 50 percent of women think heart disease is the major cause and many women are much more concerned about breast cancer. Why wouldn't they be? We see pink ribbons, bracelets, and T-shirts everywhere to "save the tatas." Even NFL players wear pink shoes and gloves every October for breast cancer awareness. Breast cancer is an awful disease to cope with and can be deadly, but we need to know that heart disease causes almost ten times the number of deaths in women.[53] The second largest cause of women's death is all types of cancer, accounting for 21 percent of all women's deaths. Of that 21 percent, the most common type of cancer to cause women's deaths is lung cancer, followed by breast cancer.[54] Race does appear to play a role in causes of death: American Hispanic women die equally from cancer and heart disease, but European-American and African-American women are more likely to die from heart disease.

While European-American women are more likely to be diagnosed with breast cancer, African-American women are more likely to die from it.[55]

## Osteoporosis

Our mothers told us to drink milk for a reason. Women accumulate calcium and bone density throughout their youth.[56] Then, five to ten years after menopause, lower estrogen levels can cause women to lose some bone density, increasing the risk for bone fractures.[57] In the first five years after menopause, women can lose from 9 to 13 percent of bone density,[58] and there are many factors that influence to what degree this will happen. Some of these are a little counterintuitive. Overweight women with a BMI of 26 to 29, and obese women with a BMI of 30 and up, are *less* likely to lose bone density after menopause than women with a BMI between 18 and 25. Women who drink alcohol moderately are also less likely to lose bone density compared to women who drink excessively and those who don't drink at all. Good news for curvy wine drinkers! Other ways to maintain bone density are more consistent with the usual recommendations for healthy living: eating fruits and vegetables, doing weight-bearing exercise like walking, and not smoking.[59] Medications like Boniva help to increase bone density, but have gastrointestinal side effects and can be costly. Estrogen replacement therapy is effective in preventing bone density loss, especially when it is started close to menopause. However, there are serious health risks and side effects, such that the medical community advises doctors to prescribe it for the shortest time possible.[60]

In terms of physical health, most women pass through this transition with minimal, manageable disturbances. How physical symptoms are experienced is influenced by decidedly nonbiological factors like cultural, racial, and generational differences. The increased risks of heart disease and osteoporosis in postmenopausal women can be effectively moderated by lifestyle choices.

In the past fifty years, popular culture has presented menopause as an inevitable decline in women's health and value that is independent of the physical symptoms they experience. These attitudes developed because of the suspicion of women's reproductive processes inherent in the hormone myth. At yet another phase of life, we can exclaim, "There go those pesky hormones again!" It's an easy, simplistic—but false—understanding of how women's bodies work. The myth that hormonal changes during menopause turn women into sickly, nagging bitches or vapid cows is just that—an empty myth. It became entrenched in medical and popular opinion because of the profit motive of pharmaceutical companies, and chauvinistic ideas of an ideal woman as perennially youthful, attractive, and compliant. In the next chapter, we will see the statistical truth: that menopausal women are not sick and sad; in fact, for most women it is a time of happy thriving.

# CHAPTER 9

# Aging Into One of the Happiest Times of Life

As is the case with many aspects of women's reproductive health, there is not a lot of research focusing on the possible positive feelings and experiences related to the menopause transition. When researchers examine a topic with a preconceived notion that there could only be negative outcomes, they structure their research to measure only negative outcomes. For example, in many studies researchers gave women a menopause symptom scale to identify possible physical and emotional problems related to menopause.[1] Few studies included something like a "menopausal happiness scale." If women felt any positive aspects of menopause, they had nowhere to report them to researchers. But that doesn't mean positive feelings don't exist.

## THE UPSIDE OF MENOPAUSE

There have been several studies that interviewed women and asked, in open-ended ways, how they experienced the menopausal years—allowing for the possibility of positive responses.[2] Women reported a remarkable number of recurring, encouraging themes about living through the menopause transition, including these common ones.

### No More Periods

Many women were very happy to not have to deal with periods anymore. No more worrying if they got a period by surprise or if they had tampons in their purses. Women who had suffered from bad cramps were happy to never have them again. For women who preferred not to have sex during their period, menopause meant that sexual satisfaction could always be on the menu.

## No Worries About Pregnancy

Most American women try to regulate when and how many times they get pregnant. While the majority use birth control during their childbearing years, there still is no perfectly reliable method without side effects or risks. Hormonal methods like the pill and the patch are very reliable but can cause a whole host of side effects like weight gain, migraine headaches, and serious health risks for smokers.[3] Nonhormonal methods like condoms and diaphragms have very few side effects but are nowhere near as effective. Menopausal women in these studies were relieved to walk away from that conundrum and to have sex with no fear of getting pregnant.

## A Time to Evaluate and Reprioritize

For many women, menopause brought the realization that life is probably more than half over. It marked a time of life when parents, and perhaps a few peers, died. That may sound sad, but the women interviewed said that these losses, while painful, helped them find a sense of what was important in their lives. The deaths spurred them to evaluate who they were and how they wanted to focus their time. This kind of reflection produced changes the women found exciting and energizing.

## Freedom to Focus on Self

The beginning of menopause often coincides with the chicks leaving the nest, although this will eventually become less common since more and more women are having children into their forties. I've discussed how the gold standard for being a good mother is to be emotionally and physically available for your children, at all times. With kids who have left home, women reported a newfound freedom to step away from the self-sacrificing and to spend time doing only things they wanted to do. No more driving to play rehearsal, or soccer games, or doctor visits, or for that piece of poster board for a project due tomorrow. Instead, many used this time to change their career track, to volunteer for causes that mattered to them, or to go back to school. As a professor, I can't tell you how much I loved my "returning students." Excited to be there, they always did the readings and engaged in lively, intelligent discussion. They weren't in the classroom because anyone expected them to be there; they were there completely because they wanted to be and it showed.

## Permission to Be Wise and Assertive

By the time they entered menopause, many women in these studies spoke of enjoying the competence their life experience brought them and the heightened levels of mastery they felt. They were more comfortable being assertive and said they were less likely to hesitate to express their opinions. Particularly in the working world, women often have to walk a fine line when it comes to the difference between being assertive and aggressive. If they don't speak up, ideas will never get heard, but if they speak up too much or too forcefully, no one likes them and they get called a bitch. These women in their menopausal years cared less about being liked, and more about being authentic and productive.

Research supports what these women convey: the majority of women in the menopausal years are in good mental health and are happy.[4] Most find menopause to be a bump in the road, or a minor inconvenience with occasional discomfort.[5] Only about 10 to 15 percent of women experience physical or emotional menopausal symptoms disturbing enough to seek treatment.[6]

# THE VAPID, DEPRESSED WOMAN WITH NOTHING GOING FOR HER

Even so, many physicians, psychologists, and people in general believe the menopause transition is a time of emotional instability and that hormones play an important role in this.[7] One significant reason may be that women are diagnosed with depression, across the lifespan, at about twice the rate of men. Professional and lay people alike can't resist the allure of a biological explanation for experiences like depression, despite the fact that no clear evidence supports a connection. The possibility of a biological gender difference is attractive because we already think of men and women as different, and because biological explanations seem to objectively and scientifically reinforce what we already think to be true.

One psychological theory to explain this difference is that men and women cope with sad feelings differently.[8] The idea is that when men feel sad, they tend to distract with activities and social interactions, which decreases the physical nature of being sad. Women tend to cope with sad feelings by ruminating on them—thinking about and considering the source of their sadness. According to the theory, this ruminating keeps women in a sad state and makes it easier to go down the road toward major depression. Several studies have found considerable support for this theory.[9]

At the same time, feminists have criticized the explanation. They suggest that there is nothing inherent in women, biologically or psychologically, that inevitably puts them at higher risk for depression. If women ruminate more than men, they argue, it's because women have been taught to be in touch with their feelings and men have not. But even more important to feminists is that women's lower social status creates many more reasons to be depressed. Women across the globe are more likely than men to live in poverty, be physically abused, suffer from sexual harassment, and live with laws that restrict freedom. Seeing women's responses to these hardships as mental illnesses is demeaning and mistakenly suggests that there must be something wrong with women rather than with the social institutions in which they live.[10]

Women's moods have been the focus of many, many studies. To truly understand this research, especially as it applies to menopausal women, I first need to describe how psychologists define the word "depression." In common conversation, when a woman says "I'm depressed," it can convey a variety of meanings: anywhere from being moody for the day to suffering from a suffocating hopelessness. In psychological research, there are basically two categories of how depression is measured. The first is referred to as "major depression." This is a woman who is depressed for at least two weeks. Her feelings of sadness, grief, disinterest in the things that used to bring her joy, and feeling unable to keep up are severe enough to threaten daily functioning. She can't feel close to her friends, doesn't feel like talking with anyone, and withdraws from the people in her life. This is the level of depression that requires treatment. For psychologists to establish that she has major depression, she needs to be evaluated by a mental health professional with a structured clinical interview.

The second form of depression researchers focus on is referred to as "depressive symptoms" or "mild depression," because the symptoms are less severe than major depression. To determine if a study participant is mildly depressed, researchers use self-report measures, which are like a quiz. A menopausal woman is given a list of statements like "I feel blue" or "I have trouble sleeping" and she rates each statement on a scale that goes from "rarely" to "most or all of the time." Based on the ratings she provides, a total score of depressive symptoms is calculated. For example, a widely used measure is the Center for Epidemiologic Studies Depression Scale (CES-D). It is a twenty-question scale and psychologists agree that a score above 16 reflects depressive symptoms that are higher than average.[11]

In the end, research shows that only about 5 to 7 percent of women suffer from an episode of major depression during the years of the menopause transition.[12] So throughout this discussion of depression, keep in mind that this experience is not relevant for the majority of women. When I talk about whether hormone change causes major depression, I am focusing on a small subset of women.

## Do We Even Feel Depressed?

In national studies of mental health that examine large populations of people, only about 12 percent of American women aged forty to fifty-nine report depressive symptoms.[13] But in studies specifically focusing on women during menopause, the portion of women reporting depressive symptoms is higher, ranging from 26 percent to 40 percent.[14] This difference in reporting of increased depressive symptomatology suggests the possibility that women having difficulties may be more interested in participating in studies about menopause than those who don't. This creates the false impression that more women are in distress during menopause.

Another issue to consider is: what does it actually mean to have elevated scores on self-report measures of depressive symptoms like the CES-D? These kinds of scales may inflate the number of women identified as depressed. Studies show that of the people who score over 16 on the CES-D—which indicates elevated depressed mood—only 30 percent actually suffer from major depression. So the assumption that women in general, and menopausal women in particular, suffer from depression at higher rates may be based on an overly sensitive means of measurement.

Agreeing with a statement on a survey like "I feel depressed" may indicate changes in mood that are not far from the normal ebb and flow of human emotions.[15]

## Do Hormones Make Us Depressed?

There are very few studies that have measured the potential effect of hormones on major depression. Not because major depression isn't an important issue, but because diagnosing it requires professional staff, takes a lot of time, and therefore costs a lot of money. When researchers are awarded grants for studies, they have to make the best use of their limited resources—which make studies using structured clinical interviews rare. Also, determining hormone levels can be a challenge because it requires women to give blood or urine samples. People don't easily volunteer, so they usually need to be paid to provide incentive using substantial grant money.

Despite these difficulties, three excellent studies examine the possible relationship of hormones and major depression. The first, called Study of Women's Mental Health Across the Nation (SWAN), followed 221 premenopausal women for ten years. Each year, researchers determined if participants had major depression and measured reproductive hormone levels with blood tests. It showed that, throughout the menopause transition, changes in hormone levels were not related to developing major depression.[16]

The second study, called the Penn Ovarian Aging Study (POAS) evaluated 436 premenopausal women for eleven years. Using methods similar to those of the SWAN study, the POAS evaluated women each year for major depression using a structured clinical interview and yearly blood tests to establish their reproductive hormone levels. It did find that changes in estradiol, which is a form of estrogen, predicted depressive symptoms and that increases in FSH predicted fewer depressive symptoms.[17] Overall, there was no association of hormone levels to a diagnosis of major depression.[18]

Another long-term study used the CES-D to assess depressive symptoms. The Seattle Midlife Women's Health Study examined 164 women over eight years and measured reproductive hormone levels and depression symptoms each year. It also showed that levels of hormones didn't influence depressive symptoms.[19]

Although only three studies explored this question, their validity is very strong, with a high number of subjects and a procedure that examined women prospectively over the menopausal transition, and they assessed the study variables with highly reliable measures. We can have confidence in the results of studies with such high-quality methods. Psychologists who have reviewed the existing research on this issue conclude that there is currently not enough evidence to support the idea that changes in reproductive hormones put a woman at risk for depressive symptoms.[20]

## Do Different Menopausal Stages Affect Depression?

Another way that researchers study women's mental health during menopause is by examining the relationship between menopausal stages and women's moods. Many studies explored this question, and again, there were conflicting results. Some studies found that being in the menopausal transition stage isn't associated with depressive symptoms. In the studies that did find an association, menopausal stage contributed only a small risk for an increase in depressive symptoms for some women.[21] Most studies also identified many other variables that have much larger influences on women's moods at this time of their lives—which have nothing to do with menopause.[22] Because of this, researchers concluded that for most women, the menopausal transition stage does not increase the risk for depressive symptoms. And for the subset of women who do feel depressed at this time of life, menopausal stage plays a small role.[23]

Since changes in hormones and menopausal stage don't figure significantly in women's mental health in midlife, what does? As I showed with PMS, pregnancy, and postpartum disorders, previous psychological history and current situational factors are bigger predictors of mental health than the biology of menopause.

## DON'T BLAME MENOPAUSE: CONSIDER THE BIGGER PICTURE

When I was young, I thought everyone over forty was old. I thought old people were sweet, sedate, not too smart or sophisticated, and definitely not sexy. Now that I am in my fifties, I have thoroughly revamped that belief—as you might imagine. But aging is tough for American women, because of the premium placed on looking and seeming young. Nora Ephron captured how hard it is to see yourself aging in her popular book *I Feel Bad About My Neck: And Other Thoughts on Being a Woman*. She writes, "If I pass a mirror, I avert my eyes. If I must look into it, I begin by squinting, so that if anything really bad is looking back at me, I am already halfway to closing my eyes to ward off the sight."

Men certainly don't have to deal with this to the degree that women do: their gray hair is "distinguished" and their age brings them an aura of wisdom and leadership. Older actors play exciting characters and get romantically paired with women decades younger. For the movie *Third Person*, perennial action star Liam Neeson, at sixty, was paired with twenty-nine-year-old Olivia Wilde. Older actresses can barely get starring roles, except for the few megastars like Helen Mirren and Meryl Streep. We don't revere the old in our culture, and women's perceived value takes the strongest hit.

Growing old in this climate can challenge even the most resilient women. Many different aspects of ourselves and our life situations dictate how well we will manage what comes with the menopausal years. Some of it we have control over, and some of it we don't. Here are the most influential situations women face at this time in their lives.

## Depression Has Been an Ongoing Struggle

As we saw with postpartum depression, the most powerful predictor of a woman feeling depressed during the menopause transition is that she has suffered from depression in the past. People who have been previously depressed are at higher risk for later episodes of depression throughout their lives, compared to those who have not.[24] A history of depression appears to reflect a higher vulnerability to having any difficulty in life affect emotions.[25]

## A Woman's Plate Can Stay Too Full

Psychologists have long known that coping with stressful situations affects well-being across the lifespan. Women in their fifties and sixties often shoulder the double duty of caring for ailing parents while still having children at home. When a parent becomes hospitalized or a teenager gets suspended from school, the responsibility to manage these events can be logistically and emotionally exhausting. Situations like this override just about everything else in determining emotions. Many studies confirm the large influence that stressful events have on depression and general well-being at this time of life.[26]

## Money Hits Home When Retirement Is on the Horizon

Anyone who has gone through a time when money was tight knows the stress and strain of financial insecurity. As women enter the menopausal years, the chances that they will have trouble making ends meet goes up. While most women work while raising a family, they often make compromises in their careers that help them cope with family responsibilities, but result in a less advantageous financial position.[27] They take time off after the birth of a child and sometimes limit work hours so they can perform the "second shift" of women's work at home. Women are also less likely to have had jobs that provide a pension. Along with the long-term consequences of the gender pay gap, these differences accumulate to put women at midlife and later at a higher risk of poverty than men.[28] The SWAN study found women in the menopausal years who said it was "very hard to pay for basics" to be at considerably higher risk for high depressive symptoms.[29]

## Empty-Nest Divorces

The menopausal transition can coincide with the time that kids leave home, and at this point, many people take stock of their marriage and find it is not what they want anymore. Divorce rates in the United States for couples over fifty have doubled in the last twenty years.[30] Under the best of circumstances, divorce is a stressful process. And under the worst, it can have a ruinous impact on emotional health. When people are asked to rate how stressful certain life events are, divorce is right up there in the top two, surpassed only by death of a spouse.[31] Getting divorced entails many emotional and logistical adjustments: coping with feelings of sadness, anger, and grief; finding a new place to live; anticipating the difficulties of rejoining the dating world; and living with a smaller budget.[32]

A woman's risk of suffering physical violence also increases, especially if she initiates the divorce.[33] When researchers study women who get divorced during the menopausal years, they find that they have generally lower feelings of well-being and are more likely to experience depressed symptoms than women who don't divorce.[34]

## The Old-Girls' Club and Networks of Support

It's no surprise that having people in a social circle who care about each other is good for mental health. There is nothing like knowing that you are loved and that you have people to share your ups and downs. In tough times, caring family and friends can lend sympathetic ears, help sort out troubles, and give tangible and intangible help. People satisfied with the social support they receive report higher feelings of self-worth, life satisfaction, and happiness than those who aren't.[35] In stressful situations they are more likely to engage in positive styles of coping, like problem-solving, than negative styles, like procrastination or getting drunk.

For someone who lacks these kinds of relationships, life can feel lonely and isolating. Feeling like you have very little support from others increases vulnerability to responding with depressed feelings when stressful events do occur.[36] Several studies find that women in the menopausal transition who don't have supportive social relationships are less likely to be happy and satisfied with their lives.[37]

Despite all this research and all the positive day-to-day experiences of menopausal women, the hormone myth has us in its grips. This is because there is great financial gain to be had in defining the menstrual transition as a time of illness that makes all women sick and sad. Now that you've seen the reality of women's positive mental health during menopause, in the next chapter, I will show how concerns for profit—rather than women's health—established a multibillion dollar industry to "treat" menopause.

# CHAPTER 10

# Be Afraid of the Menopausal Profit Monster

If most of us don't become sickly, depressed, wizened nags during menopause, who is benefitting most from spreading and maintaining the myth that we do? Like so many things in modern life, it comes down to cold, hard cash. The pharmaceutical and medical industries make enormous profits by manipulating our cultural fear of aging. Ideally, their agenda would be purely to improve people's health. But we live in a capitalist society and—while there are many advantages to this economic system in terms of creativity, motivation, and potentials for advancement and wealth—in healthcare, there are some serious disadvantages. Because the pursuit of profit overtakes patients' well-being as the most important outcome.

Pharmaceutical companies are, first and foremost, beholden to their stockholders. And an ideal way for them to profit is to create an illness that affects a large percentage of people, can only be treated by a drug the company produces, and requires a person to take the medication daily for thirty or forty years. This chapter tells the story of how hormone replacement therapy became, and remains, the motherlode of all profit streams.

## WRITING A MYTH TO PROFIT FROM IT

In chapter 8, I began the story of Ayerst Laboratories, the first company to successfully manufacture and sell estrogen that was cost-effective.[1] The drug was named Premarin, because the estrogen was extracted from pregnant mares' urine. After substantial lobbying by Ayerst, Premarin was approved by the FDA to treat *severe* symptoms of menopause, like hot flashes. This approval came despite that fact that there was already evidence that manufactured estrogen increased the risk of breast cancer. But the risks were ignored. In the 1950s and 1960s, estrogen therapy became popular to treat physical symptoms of menopause and was shown to be very effective.[2] Then in 1966, *Feminine Forever* made Robert A. Wilson's case that menopause is an estrogen-deficiency disease and that women become dried up, cow-like shrews if they don't treat that deficiency. Wilson advocated that all women—whether they had symptoms or not—should take manufactured estrogen from the time they start menopause until death. This book was widely read and excerpts were published in popular magazines like *Vogue* and *Look*.[3]

What most people didn't know was that Wilson's research was funded by Ayerst. They paid for him to write *Feminine Forever* and even helped him write it. Ayerst also financed his promotional book tour and even secretly bought enough copies of the book at retail price to maintain its bestseller status.[4]

It is shocking, but true: much of our cultural perception about menopause and aging in women was established, promoted, and maintained in order to make a profit. This is the ultimate abuse of our capacity for myth-making, as through the decades it has affected countless women's lives in such vast ways that they are impossible to quantify or even completely convey. This menopause myth purposely created disharmony between husbands and wives, held women up to impossible ideals, caused them illnesses through side effects, and drove right into the heart of their self-esteem. Wilson's myth should be counted among the causes of depression that some women experience in mid-life. And instead of attending groups to support each other through menopause, women need support groups to recover from the damage of this particularly nasty and insidious storyline about aging—as well as its cure.

## FIGHTING AGAINST PATIENT INFORMATION

By the time the 1970s arrived, hormone replacement therapy was common. Many women were convinced that with the onset of menopause, the best way to stay healthy and attractive was to take Premarin. However, there was also a rise in cases of uterine cancer among users. The *New England Journal of Medicine* reported that those taking Premarin had between four and fourteen times the increased risk of uterine cancer,[5] and that it was highest for long-term users. Several studies followed that confirmed this outcome, but Wilson was not deterred. He said the idea that estrogen caused endometrial cancer was "the worst lie in the world, the worst fallacy" because none of the doctors he collaborated with had observed any cases of cancer in patients taking estrogen.[6] I don't know if this was wishful thinking or deliberate subterfuge. Either way, it was dangerous for women. Women were taking drugs prescribed by doctors that gave them cancer. Other studies in the 1970s found that estrogen users also had a higher risk for developing breast cancer[7] and gallbladder disease.[8]

As these risks became more widely known, the number of women taking Premarin decreased. Sales of Premarin were also hurt when the FDA required Ayerst to include an information packet that warned patients of the possible carcinogenic risks. This mandate was resisted by doctors and the pharmaceutical industry. The following organizations all came together to take legal action *against* the FDA: The American Pharmaceutical Manufacturers Association, Ayerst Pharmaceuticals, The American College of Obstetrics and Gynecology, and the American Cancer Society.[9]

Wait a minute. The American Cancer Society joined litigation against distributing patient information about the risk of cancer? It makes sense that pharmaceutical industry representatives objected because "patient information would reduce sales of estrogen drugs and reduce profits."[10] But an association with the primary goal of preventing cancer? It doesn't seem to make sense, unless you understand that physicians set the agenda of the American Cancer Society—and in this case, they did not want to relinquish their monopoly on medical knowledge. Physicians opposed including information packets because doing so would reduce their autonomy to decide how much information a patient should know.[11] While we would like to think a doctor would want patients to know about such serious health risks, at that time doctors still held an authoritarian position in patient relations—and losing that authority was threatening.

There is not even a pretense of concern for women's health in this legal position and the lack of concern for women's health and well-being is painful to hear. Fortunately, the FDA prevailed and this information was made available to women. But there is so much more to the story.

# A NEW BAD GUY FOR HORMONE THERAPY TO FIGHT: OSTEOPOROSIS

Scientists discovered that by lowering the dose of estrogen and combining it with synthetic progesterone—known as *progestin*, the risk of endometrial cancer was greatly reduced. But many women had become hesitant to use hormone therapy for hot flashes and maintaining youthfulness. So, to make up for lost sales, Ayerst refocused their efforts on selling estrogen as a treatment for the loss of bone density.[12]

It was known that when women have their ovaries removed in an oophorectomy, they are thrown into an early and severe menopause, and suffer substantial bone loss. A randomized controlled study in 1982 found that after oophorectomy, women treated with a dosage of .625 mg of estrogen experienced much less bone loss than those who received a smaller dosage or no estrogen at all.[13] The results of this study addressed a very particular group of women—those who had a surgical menopause *only*. Even so, without scientific evidence, estrogen was marketed to *all* women as a "proven" way to stop bone loss. In 1986, pharmaceutical companies received approval from the FDA to claim that estrogen could treat the loss of bone density that comes with old age.[14]

Yet women still had their doubts. To get them to undertake hormone therapy again, a dire medical necessity had to be created. A massive publicity campaign was carried out by Ayerst, and messages about "deadly" osteoporosis were spread through radio, television, and magazines. The reality is that only fifteen percent of American women suffer from osteoporosis[15]—not an illness a woman is likely to develop. And if she does, she is unlikely to have the kind of fracture that is life-threatening. Breaks to the hip and the vertebrae are most highly related to an increased risk of death, but they make up very few of the fractures that people with osteoporosis experience.[16] But Ayerst publicized that every woman was at serious risk, massively overstating it. Their efforts convinced physicians and nurses to spread the word that hormone therapy could save them from this disease. A publicity firm hired nurses to run seminars for church groups and women's clubs about osteoporosis, and financed a national tour of physicians to educate the public on the danger—and the hormone therapy cure.[17] All without knowing whether or not hormone therapy was effective in preventing bone loss in women who enter menopause naturally.

Their campaign was highly successful. By the 1990s, Premarin was the most commonly prescribed medication in the United States, providing one billion dollars in sales to Ayerst—now known as Wyeth-Ayerst Laboratories. That number is particularly amazing, since only half the population was eligible to receive it and research continued to find an elevated risk of breast cancer in women who took it. All the same, ads continued to appeal to women's desires to appear young and vital, and to play off their great fear of looking old. One company ran an ad for Estraderm patch with "before" and "after" pictures. The before picture was Picasso's *Woman Dressing Her Hair,* which in the ad was meant to convey a grotesque, misshapen woman with flailing breasts. The after picture was of an ethereal, sensual, and appealing woman from Botticelli's *Primavera.*[18] Regardless of taste in art, the message being conveyed was that if you don't take hormones, you will be a disturbing interpretation of a woman, rather an ideal example of what a woman should be.

## THE WONDER DRUG GETS MORE POWERFUL: HEART DISEASE AND DEMENTIA

Sales continued to climb when experts started touting hormone therapy as a way for women to avoid not only bone loss, but also heart disease and dementia. In 1995, the *Harvard Women's Health Watch* advised confidently that "estrogen is considered to be responsible for [women's] fifteen-to-twenty-year advantage over men in evading coronary artery disease. Not only do most women have little evidence of heart problems during their reproductive years, when estrogen levels are high, but those who take estrogen after menopause seem to have lower rates of heart attack."[19] The operative word used there was "seem."

For many years, doctors had noticed   anecdotally—that patients on hormone therapy seemed less likely to develop these conditions. Several observational studies found an association between hormone therapy and decreased rates of heart disease, osteoporosis, dementia, and cognitive decline.[20] The prospect of being able to prevent dementia is powerful. There are many aspects of physical illness that are frightening, but to me, personally, nothing is as terrifying as losing my mind, my grasp on reality, and the ability to mentally function. If there was a pill to prevent that, I would take it. But observational studies are not randomized controlled studies. With observational studies, it is only possible to establish an association between a treatment and an outcome—not causation. For example, women who took hormones were more likely to have less heart disease, but that didn't mean the hormone therapy *caused* the decrease in heart disease. It's possible that women who take hormones are more focused on health issues and actually have less heart disease because they eat healthy and exercise—not because they take hormones.

The only way to find out if hormones actually cause good health outcomes for women is to do a randomized controlled study in which women are randomly assigned to a group taking hormones or to a control group taking placebos. Then, over time, their rates of heart disease, osteoporosis, and dementia would be documented. Amazingly, after fifty years of prescribing hormones to women, this type of study had *never* been done. You, your mother, your sisters, or your friends may have been taking a medication for years—even decades—that had not been rigorously tested to see if it actually does what the manufacturers said it does. Much less tested to see what, exactly, the risks of taking it are.

This lack of randomized controlled studies to support the use of hormones in preventing heart disease, osteoporosis, and dementia led the FDA to send a warning letter to Wyeth-Ayerst in 1999, expressing concerns that the company was making claims for which there was no strong scientific support. It was being used "off-label," a term that refers to prescribing drugs for conditions that have not been verified by the FDA. The FDA also expressed concerns that this widespread use was particularly troublesome because of the known cancer risks of hormone use.[21]

## IF SCIENCE PROVES CLAIMS WRONG, THEY JUST REWRITE THE MYTH

With funding from Wyeth-Ayerst, scientists finally undertook a randomized controlled study on hormones and heart disease.[22] The study was also "double-blind," because neither the experimenters nor the subjects were aware of who was assigned to the hormone therapy group or the placebo group—which helps to decrease an expectation bias. It came to be known as the HERS study, which is an acronym for The Heart and Estrogen/Progestin Replacement Study. Participants included 3,000 postmenopausal women who had already been diagnosed with heart disease. The purpose was to establish whether taking a combination of estrogen and progestin, marketed by Wyeth-Ayerst under the brand name Prempro, prevented secondary cardiovascular events like heart attacks, compared to similar women who did not take these hormones. The medical community typically gives the findings of such a rigorous study substantial weight when considering the usefulness of a particular therapy. But the results were not encouraging. After four years, the women taking Prempro did not have any fewer heart attacks than the control group; in fact, they had a slightly higher number of heart attacks. Prempro users also had more blood clots and a higher risk of developing gallbladder disease.

How did Wyeth-Ayerst respond? Did they tell doctors to stop prescribing hormone therapy to prevent heart disease? No, they did not. A few months before the study became public in 1998, Wyeth-Ayerst initiated a worldwide campaign to warn women that estrogen loss could cause dangerous consequences, and to encourage them to see their doctor about hormone therapy.[23] In spite of convincing evidence that hormone therapy didn't prevent heart-disease progression and that it caused serious health risks like blood clots and gall bladder disease, Wyeth doubled down efforts to maintain their cash cow by convincing menopausal women they had a disease—and that only a doctor and the hormones he could prescribe would protect them.

This blatant misrepresentation of the efficacy and safety of hormone therapy continued. In 2000, Wyeth-Ayerst hired glamorous model and actress Lauren Hutton as a spokeswoman. She was featured on the cover of Parade, a popular national Sunday-newspaper insert. In the interview, she said that her secret to looking and feeling young was taking estrogen. Alongside was a Wyeth-Ayerst ad that portrayed Hutton describing scary ailments estrogen loss can bring.[24] The campaign that this was a part of crystalized the misogynistic idea that looking young and desirable was just as important as being healthy, and that menopause could threaten both. It just reinforced the old notion that women are objects that must appear young and pleasing to look at—no matter the cost.

But celebrities can be tremendously influential when they bring attention to medical issues. This was well-demonstrated when, after her husband died of colon cancer, Katie Couric publicized her colonoscopy, a highly effective test to detect colon cancer early enough for treatment to be more successful. In a powerful display of personal investment, Couric had a doctor perform a colonoscopy on her during the widely seen *Today* show. In the following years, the number of Americans getting this test went up by 20 percent, undoubtedly saving lives.[25]

Hutton's campaign with Wyeth-Ayerst was powerful as well. Up until 2001, Prempro was one of their top-selling drugs. But rather than improve women's lives, it again cemented the myth of menopause as a medical disease rather than a natural stage of reproductive health. It encouraged women to take a drug just when evidence that it was ineffective and dangerous was piling up. Even as the HERS study used impressively rigorous methods and a subject pool of 3,000 women, an even more powerful study was underway.

# RESCUED BY THE WOMEN'S HEALTH INITIATIVE

To women's health activists of the 1980s and 1990s, one of the most important issues they tackled was the practice of excluding women as participants in the majority of medical studies. Researchers were concerned that women's menstrual cycles would complicate study results, making it more difficult to establish the effectiveness of a drug or treatment. This meant that broad generalizations about disease, treatment, and prevention were applied to women, based on research only done on men.[26] As a result, women weren't benefitting from biomedical research.

To address this dearth of research on women, Representatives Patricia Schroeder and Henry Waxman, along with Senator Olympia Snowe, advocated for institutional change in how studies were funded and carried out. The National Institutes of Health (NIH), the government agency that controls much of the country's budget for medical research, received substantial funding for research to increase knowledge of women's health. Bernadine Healy, MD, became the first female director of the NIH in 1991 and introduced plans for the Women's Health Initiative (WHI)—an important step in government sponsorship of methodologically strong research on women's health. More than 150,000 women at forty research centers across the nation were included in a group of studies on the causes of illness and death in older women.

One of those studies was a double-blind, randomized controlled study of hormone use in about 27,000 postmenopausal women aged between fifty and seventy-nine. Women were randomly assigned to groups that received Premarin (estrogen), Prempro (estrogen plus progestin), or a placebo. The plan was to evaluate the women regularly over a fifteen-year period to measure the effect of hormone therapy on the three major outcomes for which hormone therapy was being prescribed as a preventative: heart disease, dementia, and hip fractures. The prevalence of a variety of negative health outcomes, like breast cancer and stroke, was also to be evaluated.[27] This study had impressive financial and logistical commitments to using the highest quality research. The hopes were high that the medical community would finally obtain a reliable answer as to whether or not hormone therapy was the panacea so many doctors and pharmaceutical companies had promised for so long. The results of the study were beyond shocking: researchers found that hormone therapy was so bad for women that the only ethical thing to do was to stop the study early.

The clinical trial of women taking Prempro or a placebo was shut down after only five years because women taking Prempro—compared to the women taking placebos—had a 29 percent *increased* rate of cardiovascular events like heart attacks; a 26 percent *higher* rate of breast cancer; a 41 percent *increase* in strokes; and a 100 percent *increase* in dementia. They did, however, experience fewer fractures and increased their bone mass density.[28] The clinical trial of women taking Premarin or a placebo was shut down in 2004 because the women in the Premarin group had higher rates of dementia and stroke compared to women taking placebos. Premarin did not cause an increased risk of heart disease, breast cancer, colorectal cancer, or blood clots, and was responsible for a lower incidence of hip fractures.[29]

These results compelled the FDA to require a black box warning, which is its most severe warning and is designed to call attention to serious or life-threatening risks,[30] on Prempro and drugs like it. These warnings plainly stated that estrogen and progestin shouldn't be prescribed to prevent heart disease and clearly documented that the WHI had found that women who took estrogen and progestin had higher risks of having heart attacks and strokes, and developing invasive breast cancer, pulmonary embolism, and deep vein thrombosis.[31]

The manufacturer of Prempro and Premarin, now known as Wyeth, had annual sales of $2.5 billion before the WHI trials were stopped.[32] Just take that number in for a moment. Two-and-a-half-billion dollars every year. That stratosphere sheds some light on the things a company would do to maintain it. After the WHI hormone therapy trials ended, Wyeth's financial picture changed within one year. Due to cratering revenue from hormone therapy drugs and because they needed to set aside $2 billion to cover lawsuits due to heart damage, Wyeth reported a quarterly loss of $426.4 million and stock prices dropped from fifty dollars to thirty-four dollars and fifty cents.[33] Doctors went back to prescribing hormone therapy for only the short-term relief of menopausal symptoms like hot flashes and vaginal dryness.

## WHO'S INFLUENCING YOUR DOCTOR'S TREATMENT MOST?

As appalling as it is that pharmaceutical companies willfully and aggressively compromised women's health to make a profit, it is not unfathomable since the first priority of any company is to make money. But what about the doctors who prescribe such treatments? Doctors aren't idealized and put on a pedestal the way they used to be, but most people still presume their doctors have the health of their patients as a guiding purpose in any medical practice. And I'm sure that many do. But there is a tangled financial connection between doctors and pharmaceutical companies that compromises this goal.

Anyone who has sat in the waiting room at a doctor's office knows there is often an extremely attractive and well-dressed person who gets to see the doctor first: the pharmaceutical rep. Their role, ostensibly, is to keep the doctor informed on the latest news about medications and treatments produced by their company. But they also come with free drug samples. Since health insurance and medications are so expensive, patients love free samples, and I understand that doctors can want to give their patients that break. Pharmaceutical reps also regularly bring platters of food for the whole medical staff. In 2005, *Annals of Family Medicine* published a powerful entreaty for doctors to refuse to see these reps. Its review of empirical data shows "that interactions with pharmaceutical reps increase the chances that the physician will act contrary to duties owed to the patient."[34]

Doctors also receive funds from pharmaceutical companies to support their research, and get paid to do speaking engagements and to provide consulting.[35] Does getting paid by a drug company influence the way doctors represent their drugs? There are many studies that suggest it does.[36] A study particularly relevant to this discussion showed how this conflict of interest can play out. It examined opinion pieces on the results of the WHI study—letters, editorials, and comments—that appeared in medical journals between 2002 and 2006. In spite of the convincing evidence provided by the WHI, 64 percent of the articles criticized the WHI and promoted the use of hormone therapy. It turned out that a core group of ten doctors had authored four or more articles each, accounting for a large percentage of the total articles that appeared on this topic. Eight of the ten doctors had received payment for speaking or consulting from hormone therapy manufacturers. In general, articles promoting the treatment of menopause with hormone therapy were 2.4 times as likely to have been written by a doctor who had been paid by hormone manufacturers.[37]

This kind of misrepresentation is dangerous because it serves to shape the opinions of medical practitioners. As recently as 2008, about half of American gynecologists report that they distrust the findings of the WHI.[38] And this unfounded doubt reaches patients seeking information about hormone therapy. If you visit WebMD looking for information about the benefits and risks of hormone therapy, the website still describes the WHI findings as "controversial."[39] They might have been a shock for Wyeth stockholders, but scientifically there is nothing controversial about them.

When the findings of the WHI became public, many women stopped taking hormones like Premarin and Prempro, but those with disturbing menopausal symptoms continued to seek relief. A new industry with bioidentical hormones stepped in to fill that need.

## BIOIDENTICAL HORMONES REPEAT THE SAME STORY

Actress Suzanne Somers is best known for her role in the early 1980s sitcom *Three's Company* as the blonde and beautiful, but ditzy, Chrissy

Snow. At the age of fifty-eight, looking remarkably young, Somers began a second career by endorsing the hormone myth for the new millennium and promoting bioidentical hormones as a cure for menopause. Her 2004 book on the topic was titled *The Sexy Years,* and in it she tells readers that after encountering the "seven dwarfs of menopause—Itchy, Bitchy, Sweaty, Sleepy, Bloated, Forgetful, and All-Dried-Up," she found the fountain of youth. Somers promises that bioidentical hormone therapy will help menopausal women lose weight and fight the symptoms of aging. Here, and also in the follow-ups *Ageless* and *I'm Too Young for This,* she tells readers that the drop in reproductive hormones that comes with menopause gives women "murderous moods" and "robs them of their lives." The books all have covers that show Somers looking smooth and wrinkle-free, telegraphing the thought that, if only you took these drugs, you also could look young into your sixties. This is despite the fact that much of Somer's smooth skin appears to come from Botox, fillers, and plastic surgery (nobody has lips that get fuller as they age, nobody). Her experience, and those of the women she interviewed, are the basis for her claims—with scant scientific evidence.

The bioidentical hormone therapy Somers promotes refers to hormones extracted from plants rather than horses. They are produced by compounding pharmacies based on a physician's specific prescription for that patient, and because bioidentical hormone compounds are created with varying levels of hormones, they are not regulated by the FDA. They are marketed as "bioidentical" because of manufacturer claims that they are chemically and structurally identical to the hormones produced by women. There is no scientific evidence to currently support this claim and the FDA does not recognize the term.[40]

Bioidentical hormones are marketed as a safe alternative to traditionally prescribed hormones. Somers and the pharmacies selling these products promise that bioidentical hormones will protect women from cancer, heart disease, and Alzheimer's disease, and will also return the lean, shining bodies of their youth.[41] Sound familiar? These are the same magical claims Wyeth-Ayerst made about traditional hormone therapy. And the financial potential is, once again, huge. Estimates of annual sales suggest compounded bioidentical hormones account for a multibillion dollar industry.[42]

What we know for sure about bioidentical hormones is what we have always known about forms of estrogen and progesterone: they ease physical symptoms of menopause like hot flashes. There are many studies that support this conclusion and the FDA has approved a few types of these plant-based hormones for this specific purpose. But the bioidentical hormones approved by the FDA are different from compounded bioidentical hormones, because the dosage and contents of those with FDA approval are standardized rather than personalized. There is also some evidence that bioidentical hormones may prevent bone density loss in postmenopausal women.[43] But scientifically speaking, that is all we know. Very few long-term, randomized controlled studies have examined these drugs, therefore it is unknown if bioidentical hormones protect against heart disease or dementia.

Even more importantly, we don't know whether these drugs carry the same risks as traditional hormones. While it is possible that bioidentical hormones are safe and effective, we currently don't have the scientific evidence to support that claim—a few encouraging studies is not enough. The WHI taught us that when physicians prescribe drugs for women without appropriate testing, they expose us to unnecessary risks. This is why seven doctors wrote an open letter to Suzanne Somers and her publisher that elaborates on all the ways they "believe *Ageless* is detrimental and dangerous to the thousands of women who read it because the book freely and repeatedly blurs the line of medical ethics and science with hearsay." The doctors who signed this letter include three who were quoted in Somers's book and five who have written popular books on menopause, including Dr. Christiane Northrup.[44]

Women need accurate information and solid science to make intelligent decisions about their health. To do that, we need to overcome the power the hormone myth has over us. By creating and marketing the myth that menopausal women are sick and in need of treatment, the medical and pharmaceutical industries failed women. With disregard for women's health, doctors prescribed hormone replacement therapy for decades without scientific evidence of its efficacy or safety. Pharmaceutical companies repeatedly marketed it as a cure-all fountain of youth. When the studies of the WHI revealed that hormone replacement therapy didn't prevent heart disease or dementia, and caused increased rates of breast cancer, heart disease, and strokes in women who used it, the damage done to women was horrifyingly clear. Financial relationships between doctors and pharmaceutical companies compromised the ability of both to provide women with treatments that put our health first. And they have given us great cause to be alert and suspicious going forward.

This is sadly yet another story in a book filled with examples of the mythic lies told to women about our health. The hormone myth has seduced us, and it's costing us big.

# CHAPTER 11

# How Lies Persist and What We Lose by Believing Them

The hormone myth's staying power and resistance to change are undeniable. Like every other theory of female inferiority down through the ages, the hormone myth sustains the patriarchal system most of humanity lives under. Men have more economic, social, and political power than women in most societies. Keeping up beliefs that men are biologically different in ways that make them better suited to have power is central to maintaining that dominance. Once power is established and supported by social, political, and economic forces—and by culture, custom, and blind habit—it tends to stay established. And so the system perpetuates the myth and the myth supports the system in a feedback loop that's really hard to break. Individually, we make choices that support it, and researchers in social psychology offer insight into why.

## HOW BELIEFS CAN CONTRADICT EXPERIENCE

People can perform amazing mental gymnastics that allow them to hold beliefs contrary to their experience. There are ways that we rationalize illogical thinking, which can be used to maintain the hormone myth as a whole,[1] which include the following.

### Illusory Optimism

People tend to believe that we are luckier or less vulnerable than others. A menopausal woman who is not depressed, may still believe that most menopausal women are depressed, but that she is one of the lucky ones who doesn't suffer.

## Self-Serving Bias

We like to believe that we are better than others. A woman who doesn't suffer from PMS might think that most women do get it, but that she is made of stronger stuff.

## False Uniqueness

Human beings also tend to believe that we are unique, when most people really are like everyone else in many ways. However, a pregnant woman who doesn't experience mood swings may think that most pregnant women will cry at the drop of a hat, but that she must be different, special in this way.

The bottom line is that in our efforts to make sense of the world, human beings make errors in their thinking. We doubt the weight of our personal experience when contrary evidence seems to be coming at us from all directions. The hormone myth is sustained by our inability to reconcile the tsunami of information that says that women are at the mercy of their hormones with the personal reality of consistently stable emotional functioning.

# WHEN WHAT EVERYBODY KNOWS ABOUT HORMONES IS NOT TRUE FOR YOU

Before I dive into an in-depth discussion about how the hormone myth is a form of gender policing—both the internal kind and the kind we enforce on each other—I want to show you how this myth can possibly persist when we're actually, statistically, not experiencing the symptoms it says we are. To do this, I'll revisit the myth as it relates to PMS, pregnancy, postpartum depression, and menopause.

## PMS Moodiness

According to the current definition of PMDD, 3 to 8 percent of American women have serious mood changes in relation to periods that are so severe they disrupt lives and relationships. Which also means that 92 to 97 percent of American women are *not* so afflicted. An indeterminate number of women—probably most women—experience mild physical and emotional changes around their periods. Various studies of PMS have identified over 150 different, possible symptoms—a number so huge as to be nearly meaningless—and the reported symptoms vary by culture. But what is *not* happening, except in very few cases, is a mental disorder tied to the menstrual cycle. Women's moods are no more changeable or extreme than men's moods. We are not all crazy once a month. It's a myth. So why would we believe something that opposes our lived experience?

It is tempting for a woman to embrace the myth of near-universal PMS because it helps her maintain the "good woman" image of always fulfilling her feminine roles happily—except when she can't help it because of her awful, awful hormones. Invoking PMS has this instant impact. *Everybody knows* it's overwhelming, overpowering, and not her fault. It offers a pass to temporarily be angry or irritable, and to otherwise flout expectations. She can break the rules without threatening the status quo.

But still, we all know the world is full of women going mad once a month. Of course, if a woman we care about tells us she's suffering, we'll tend to believe her. But maybe—and maybe more often—we assign PMS to another woman without any real evidence. Maybe she's impatient, or irritable, or easily upset, and we are labeling her according to the myth. It's entirely possible that we've bought the myth, but we believe it doesn't apply to us—which can make us feel special, unique, even superior. Women use the hormone myth and thereby keep it going. But most of us have never experienced anything extreme in tandem with our periods. Plenty of us hardly feel a blip.

## Collective Pregnancy Care

A pregnant belly triggers the hormone myth powerfully. Most people know that hormones increase to facilitate a pregnancy and believe that they instigate pretty much everything a pregnant woman does or feels. The hormone myth includes our notion of "baby brain," which evokes an image of the flighty, distracted, and emotionally irrational woman. But most mothers-to-be are in quite good mental health and perform cognitive tasks involving memory and problem solving without any trouble. So why would so many women themselves buy into this myth?

In the same way that PMS gives women permission to be angry or emotionally unavailable, the hormone myth provides women with breathing room to feel overwhelmed by all the massive changes that are happening in their lives. They get relief from feeling like they have to always be on top of everything; they get coddled in ways that can feel as good as annoying. When they can blame baby brain, they don't have to take the extreme stressors they face seriously, which include doing the majority of housework and dodging rampant discrimination at work. If a woman is unable to keep all the balls in the air—and really, no one is able to keep all those balls in the air *all* the time—baby brain becomes a reasonable excuse that is blame-free.

## Postpartum Depression Stigma

For women who suffer from postpartum depression, the hormone myth brings particularly serious consequences. In chapter 7, I described the many reasons why some women suffer from postpartum depression—previous history of depression or mental illness, lack of support with childcare, and marital conflict—and none of them have much to do with hormones. But here the hormone myth is dangerous because embedded in the ideas that women are ruled by their hormones, and that hormones cause postpartum depression, is the idea that these feelings will just pass. When depressed mothers don't get help because of this and their depression is prolonged, their health and the development of their children suffer. Women also resist getting help for postpartum depression because of the stigma attached to it. The basis of the hormone myth is that women are biologically more nurturing than men, and therefore should be natural mothers. This is what "everyone knows." But the reality is that mothering doesn't always come naturally or easily, and doesn't give every woman feelings of pleasure, is in direct opposition to this standard. Women can self-police when they deny this reality and feel too much shame to discuss it, much less ask for help. With postpartum depression, the hormone myth hurts those who *do* experience it.

## Menopausal Shifts

Seeing menopause as a sickness to be cured is a cultural way of worshipping youth and subservience in women. During menopause, a couple of things happen simultaneously: women develop confidence and assertiveness in speaking their minds, and start putting their interests ahead of others for perhaps the first time in their adult lives. These are logical changes that result from the accumulated wisdom that life experience provides, and the simple logistics of children leaving home. But when we have, for so long, bought into the agreeable, accommodating, other-focused model of good wife and mother that the hormone myth trades in—we can feel guilty or even lost. Because women are taught to fulfill this model and men are taught to expect this model.

My mother taught me how to care for a sick child with tenderness, to create wonderful Thanksgiving meals, and to put my needs last. There is satisfaction to be had in such emotional and tangible giving. When I was able to soothe one of my kids with the flu, or see people truly enjoy a meal at my table, I felt real happiness. But I've reached the age where my children have left the house and I want to focus more on my needs and interests. But the hormone myth says that if I want to do that, I'm sick, my hormones are supposedly out of whack, and I need treatment. Hormones have nothing to do with this shift in focus. It is a developmentally appropriate change. However, when women look to step out of the roles that they are biologically "meant" for even a little bit, they face resistance in many forms: from family and spouses who have gotten used to such selfless care, and sometimes even judgment from other women who continue to fulfill their gender-assigned roles so completely. It's really hard to reconceive ourselves and our places in life beyond this.

## TRAPPED BY BIOLOGY?

The hormone myth draws power from beliefs that we take for truths. In particular, *biological essentialism* is the belief that men and women are fundamentally different psychologically and behaviorally because of their different reproductive systems. Psychologists have found that we tend to exaggerate both the differences of people in different groups and the similarities of those within a group. *Gender polarization* is the tendency to perceive the most relevant difference between people to be gender.[2] So we divide people into different groups based on their reproductive organs, and then concentrate on finding similarities within groups, and differences between groups, that go far beyond the facts of reproduction. From there, our ideas about what individual people "are" and what they "should be," based on their sex, become fused into gender stereotypes and gender rules. This includes the standards of the good woman, the good mother, and the good female employee.

It's important to note that the stereotyped masculine box of rational, aggressive, and emotionless is just as restricting as the stereotyped feminine box of nurturing, happy, refined, and emotional. We are all born experiencing a broad range of emotions and personality traits, yet we put so much into teaching boys to "take it like a man" and girls to "act like a lady." I cannot imagine how much mental and emotional energy it takes for boys and men to learn to swallow their "softer" emotions and maintain a strong, manly exterior. Even though I do know how profoundly hard I worked to suppress my anger.

Men as a group benefit more from gender stereotypes in general, but they also carry some of the cost of this wasteful, dysfunctional, and even dehumanizing agreement. The never-ending pressure on men to be successfully employed, in a landscape where that's often not realistic, is enormous and relentless. And throughout history, men have paid the price of having to carry out the brutalizing work of war and risk losing their own lives. So while women have been trapped in the home, men have been trapped on the front lines of supporting the family. I want to emphasize this in the discussion that follows to show that gender-based myths, like those about women's hormones, hurt men also. Because biological essentialism is a trap that only wounds us more as we try to wriggle our way out, because it is locked shut by cultural norms. With its strength, no one can be and express the entirety of what it is to be a human being.

## THE PSYCHOLOGY BEHIND GENDER STEREOTYPING

Stereotypes aren't just about gender, of course. Human beings use stereotypes all the time, and they have a function: generalizations help us cope with all the information that comes at us every day. To function in our daily lives, we need to quickly categorize information and either drop it or store it. We conceptualize reality as simpler than it is, because our brains would get stuck if we tried to consider the full, complex nature of everything we come in contact with. Our ability to generalize and categorize is essential, and it's a strength. However, when it comes to broadly categorizing people by gender, the feature becomes a bug. Because if the category becomes more important than the people assigned to it, people suffer.

So why do we cling to gender categories even when they hurt us? Psychologists have proposed a number of theories to explain the staying power of beliefs in essential gender differences. The feminist psychoanalytic framework of Nancy Chodorow explores how children come to perceive gender roles as cornerstones of their personal identities. Albert Bandura's social learning theory, which I find particularly compelling, theorizes that people learn to have certain attitudes and behaviors if they are socially rewarded for them. Conversely, people learn to refrain from certain attitudes and behaviors if they are socially punished for them. There are many studies that support the power of rewards and punishment in enforcing attitudes and behavior.[3] Who does all this punishing and rewarding? *Socializing agents* like parents, peers, and the media all contribute to produce children and ultimately adults who accept that males and females are different, and are highly invested in "performing their gender well"[4]—that is, in being seen as "a real man" or "a real woman." When, in fact, they are simply playing along in a cultural game.

Each of these socializing agents has played a major role in maintaining the hormone myth and have all been integral to my discussion of the ways the myth plays out in women's reproductive events. I want to describe them further so that you are even better armed to recognize them for what they are: powerful influences that shape our experiences of life and ourselves.

## Shaming Parents

Parents play an active role in teaching gender to their children, but appear to have the most influence by what they teach children *not* to do.[5] Parents do tend to assign gender-typical chores, and often encourage their children to have gender-typical interests and activities. But what parents are even more likely to do is to *discourage* "gender-inappropriate" play, especially when fathers interact with sons.

During my daughter's third birthday party, a little boy picked up her *101 Dalmatians* pocketbook and proudly strolled around with it. His father sternly yelled "Josh, put that bag down now! I mean it: right now!"

It was as though the purse was a loaded gun. His father's reaction told Josh two things: that his father was angry at him, and that his father was frightened for him. I could imagine the powerful shame and fear rocketing through his little body and mind at that moment.

Many fathers are strongly concerned with keeping their sons from showing any feminine tendencies, a concern that has a lot to do with our culture's deep-rooted homophobia—the fear is that a young boy who is interested in "girly" activities is going to be gay, and the belief is that this would be a calamity. Girls acting like tomboys get more of a pass, which is in line with our increased flexibility on what is appropriate behavior for girls,[6] but only up to a point. There are some parents who resist gender-stereotyping their children, but it's a definite challenge in this pink-and-blue world. Because outside the inner family circle are our children's peers, our own peers, the marketplace, and the media.

## Punishing Peers

From a very young age, children punish violations of expected gendered behavior in other children.[7] When one of my daughters was little, she loved building things with blocks at home. But when she did this in preschool, it was with boys, because that's who played with blocks. She was quickly made fun of for playing "boy games." The pressure of this internal and external policing is as exhausting for boys and men as it is for girls and women. This gender policing continues into adolescence, and it intensifies.

Sociologist Michael Kimmel analyzed how teenage boys police each other's behavior in his disturbing book, *Guyland: The Perilous World Where Boys Become Men*. He describes the efforts that go into maintaining a masculine image and the punishments that come with failing.

> Our efforts to maintain a manly front cover everything we do. What we wear. How we talk. How we walk. What we eat (like the recent flap over "manwiches"—those artery-clogging massive burgers, dripping with extras). Every mannerism, every movement contains a coded gender language. What happens if you refuse or resist? What happens if you step outside the definition of masculinity? Consider the words that would be used to describe you. In workshops it takes generally less than a minute to get a

list of about twenty terms that are at the tip of everyone's tongues: faggot, dork, pussy, loser, wuss, nerd, queer, homo, girl, gay, skirt, Mama's boy, pussy-whipped. This list is so effortlessly generated, so consistent, that it composes a national well from which to draw epithets and put-downs.[8]

## Media Outrage

Media outlets like movies, television, and news reporting all provide examples of how people who stay within their assigned gender roles are rewarded—action hero saves the world and gets the girl, and those who don't are punished—woman doesn't wear makeup and dresses plainly so doesn't get the boy. But gender policing is never so strong as it is in the world of sports.

Mets second baseman Daniel Murphy took three days of paternity leave in 2014—as is allowed by Major League Baseball—to be with his wife and newborn son. Radio host and former NFL star Boomer Esiason criticized Murphy as neglecting his commitment to the team. Esiason said "I wouldn't do that. Quite frankly, I would have said 'C-section before the season starts. I need to be at Opening Day. I'm sorry, this is what makes our money, this is how we're going to live our life, this is going to give my child every opportunity to be a success in life.'"[9] There was only one version of manliness allowed here: breadwinner. And apparently a man who decides how and when his wife will deliver. There was no consideration for how Murphy might want to bond with his new baby, or how his wife and baby's health might be the most important factor in determining how and when she delivered—not his work schedule. It is encouraging to note that Esiason faced criticism from many people in response to his comments and he eventually apologized.

## Berating Ourselves

According to social learning theorists, after years of such reward for gender-appropriate behaviors and punishment for gender-violating behaviors, people no longer need to be policed by others because we develop internal policing. We internalize gender standards and self-regulation to maintain those standards.[10] This helps to explain why women and men, who may experience themselves as having a much wider range of attributes and interests than traditional gender roles would suggest, subscribe to these regulations. The crux is that humans are social animals. Our needs for social acceptance and validation are as basic as our needs for shelter and physical safety. When the rules are spelled out so plainly and so regularly from such a wide range of sources, it is difficult to reject them—even if our personal reality is different, and even if the rules cost us in the realms of work and personal relationships.

These cultural myths do cost us. As I hope the preceding chapters show, the losses for an individual woman can be high and, more generally, the economic and social costs for women in general are staggering. But the irony is that the hormone myth, and the ideas, theories, and habits that support it, cost men too. At its core, the basis of the hormone myth is not just that women are made emotional and irrational because of their hormones, but that they make women more emotional and irrational *than men*. By setting up women as emotional and men as unemotional, we create a lifelong imperative for men to keep their feelings repressed, suppressed, and hidden.

I mentioned in chapter 9 that women are diagnosed with depression at twice the rate of men, but a telling statistic is that men are two to three times more likely than women to abuse illicit drugs, both illegal and prescription.[11] One explanation for this is that women are socialized to feel comfortable with being emotional and asking for help. Perhaps men feel the same amount of sad emotions as women, but abusing drugs is a way for men to ease these feelings without violating the rules of masculinity. The hormone myth sets suffocating boundaries around the emotions a man can acceptably express so that he does not appear feminine.

So why do we keep paying the price? Individually and collectively, we make choices that support it—many of them based on assumptions we're not even aware of, as all this research into social psychology demonstrates. Those unexamined choices and assumptions mean that we buy, sell, and enforce the myth in our workplaces, personal relationships, and politics. Here are the major effects of doing so.

## ERODING POWER IN ANY FIELD

The research is clear: when employers and coworkers hold gender stereotypes, they can undercut worker attitudes, performance, and career choices. There is a substantial body of research which shows that when one person has stereotypical expectations of another person, those expectations can cause the other person to act in ways that will confirm the stereotype.[12] It's not magic, it has to do with what psychologists call *stereotype threat*.[13] It works this way—let's say a woman is about to take a driving test. Before she pulls out to start, the evaluator makes a crack like "Oh boy, not another woman driver." This reminder of the stereotype of women as bad drivers—despite all evidence of a contrary reality—makes her anxious and causes her to perform badly. Confidence is an important component of performance, and when that is undermined by spoken assumptions that "people like you" aren't good at this, it is hard not to be affected.

One study of gender stereotype threat illustrates how it works even when *someone else is not reminding you of the stereotype.* The erosion of confidence can happen simply when a woman is reminded that she is a "woman." In 2015, an experiment was conducted with twenty-nine female and twenty-seven male college students majoring in business, the majority of which were employed. The participants were told they were filling out a survey on their management skills, management outlook, and career aspirations. They were asked to "Rate your leadership skills" and told to estimate "How others rate your leadership skills." They also rated the degree to which they agreed with statements like "I take responsibility for my own success" and "I have dreams of being an entrepreneur." In the experimental group, participants were first asked their gender before filling out the management survey. In the control group, the management questions were asked first.

Women who were asked their gender first rated their own estimation of their management and leadership skills, and how they thought others rated them, lower than the women who were not asked. They were also substantially less likely to agree with the statements "I take responsibility for my own success" and "I have dreams of being an entrepreneur" than women who had not been reminded they were women. For the male participants, there were no differences in their responses whether they were asked their gender before the survey or not.[14]

Stereotype threat can make women question their career goals, and even change career paths.[15] Let's say a woman goes to medical school and sails through with stellar grades. When it is time to decide on a specialty, she is attracted to general surgery because she is fascinated by how the body responds to surgical treatment, and enjoys the taking apart and putting back together of the puzzle of surgery. When she has had the opportunity to participate in surgery, her advisors have praised her precision and "good hands."

However, doctors specializing in surgery are predominantly male. Surgeons have the reputation of being necessarily aggressive and arrogant. The operating idea is that in order to cut into the human body, one has to be exceptionally cold-blooded and extremely confident because any error has severe consequences. Our young female medical student finds herself to be none of these things, and doesn't see how she will fit into this culture and succeed as a surgeon. She decides to specialize in pediatrics, which is a specialty more in line with what gender stereotypes imply that women are good at. It's a specialty that is "increasingly female," as two-thirds of pediatric residents are women.[16]

You might be thinking, why does this matter? She still gets to be a doctor, and pediatricians play an important role in health care. Yes, they do, but they also make a much lower annual salary than surgeons: $189,000 versus $317,000.[17] And we know what a difference like that can have over time in creating personal wealth. There's a social cost, too: there are a limited number of people who can excel at surgery, and here is one less, fully capable person filling that role. Because of her internalized idea that she, as a woman, lacks the necessary aggressive nature, she has removed herself from a specialty that could have been greatly satisfying and highly lucrative.

People who are members of a group that is stereotyped as lacking the necessary skills to excel in a task may disengage from that entire domain.[18] It's a self-protective response—no one wants to be thought of as incompetent. So it's easier to say "I wasn't really interested in that anyway" than to face the stereotype threat. For a few years I was the executive director of a program to support female college students majoring in science, technology, engineering, and mathematics (STEM) fields, in which there is a very low percentage of women. It was plain to see that the women in the most difficult position were those in engineering. These young women found themselves in classrooms where they were the only three women among one hundred men. Visually, they appeared to not belong there, and male students and professors could be hostile. We know that women in these majors end up switching to more "female appropriate" majors like psychology or English, than men do. They disengage entirely from STEM fields; at every stage of a career, women are more likely to quit than men.[19] Part of this is that women find themselves stuck between gendered expectations at home—still doing most of the household management and childcare—and a "masculine" workplace that doesn't acknowledge these competing priorities. But a big contributor is simply a self-protective impulse. The combined pressure of dealing with a very male culture and having to represent all women with the quality of their work becomes exhausting. They abandon an entire career in which they could have made important contributions and achieved great successes.

## HOME HOLDS THE MESSAGE CLOSE

The gender stereotypes that are part and parcel of the hormone myth clearly hurt women's performance and opportunity in the workplace, but they also have a profound impact on our closest relationships. The influence of gender stereotypes on women's relationships has been most commonly studied within the context of heterosexual marriage. Among other things, these studies have found that when a husband has traditional gender attitudes he is less likely to contribute meaningfully to household duties[20] and spends fewer hours caring for their children.[21] Such men also become less satisfied with their marriage if their wives become financially independent.[22] Many studies find that when a woman has a higher income than her husband, or a more prestigious job, she is at a higher risk for physical abuse—particularly if the husband holds traditional gender attitudes.[23] On the other hand, men who hold egalitarian attitudes view their wives' paid employment as normal and worthwhile[24] and are more supportive and accommodating of their wives' work schedules.[25]

Gender stereotypes also affect how couples deal with conflict resolution. Inherent in the belief of biological essentialism is the assumption that men, because of their purported rational qualities, are better suited to hold more decision-making power in a marriage (with no hormones getting in the way). People who subscribe to traditional gender roles believe that, while women have an indispensable role to play, there can only be one head of the household, and that should be the husband. But some conflict in a marriage is inevitable. Interestingly, what is most strongly related to overall marital satisfaction is not the content of conflict—like finances, chores, or childcare—but the way in which a couple deals with conflict.

When examining conflict resolution between people, psychologists have categorized two types of strategies: *harsh* and *soft*. A person who uses harsh strategies to convince her spouse to do what she wants will do things like: become angry, threaten to do something unpleasant if the spouse doesn't agree, emphasize her legitimacy as decision-maker, or recall something unpleasant previously done by the spouse. A person who uses soft strategies will do things like: express appreciation if the other spouse agrees with him, express disappointment if they won't agree, and talk about common goals and needs.[26] A study of seventy-eight married, heterosexual couples found that husbands with a traditional gender-role ideology were more likely to use harsh conflict resolution tactics compared to husbands with a liberal gender-role ideology. And not surprisingly, when harsh tactics were used, marital satisfaction suffered. Another interesting finding in this study is that traditionally-minded couples reported more dissatisfaction when their spouse's behavior stepped outside of usual gender norms.[27]

It makes sense that the hormone myth plays an important role in such a relationship. As we've seen, people in general—and biological essentialists in particular—define a good woman as one who is always loving, caring, and available. When a wife acts outside of that ideal and expresses anger, it is likely to be especially distressing to a husband with traditional gender values. If he responds to her anger by attributing it to some kind of hormonal change, he conveys that her anger is invalid and inappropriate. And she may readily accept this, because it makes it possible for her to keep her good woman identity.

But what does that mean for the actual cause of her anger? It gets buried. Conditions that make her angry don't get addressed, whether it's always cooking as well as cleaning up after family dinners, or the lack of support she feels in disciplining the children. Conceptualizing women's anger as an unpleasant anomaly takes away any chances for her to bring positive changes to her life. It also diminishes her basic humanity, as one who has legitimate needs that deserve to be heard and considered. Sweeping women's concerns under the hormonal rug also keeps the relationship from growing. Most people change to some degree over time, and their preferences and desires may change also. In healthy relationships, adjustments are made along the way so that each person's needs are satisfied to at least some degree, if they can be. If there is never a forum to discuss or acknowledge changing needs, growth for the individual and the couple is stunted, and marital satisfaction can suffer.

## THE POLITICAL POWER PLAY

In earlier chapters, I described how the hormone myth has been used to deny women's political rights across the board. Women have always had less political power than men at every level of American government. The percentage of women holding political office has improved somewhat in the past thirty years, but it is still deplorably low considering that women make up 50 percent of the electorate. As of 2016, there are only six female governors. Women hold about 20 percent of the seats in the Senate and the House of Representatives, and about 25 percent in state legislatures.[28] In the United States, the argument that women are biologically and fundamentally different from men—too delicate, too emotional, not intelligent or aggressive enough—has kept them from the right to vote, hold political office, serve on the supreme court, or be president of the country. *Sixty-three* other countries have elected females to lead their governments.[29] The narrow gender stereotypes inherent in the hormone myth keep the number of American women in government low in several ways.

### The Likeability or Competence Conundrum

In traditional gender roles, women are and should be nurturing and kind, and men are and should be work-oriented and competitive.[30] In politics, this model puts women in an impossible double bind.[31] When a woman presents herself as assertive and competent, people are more likely to judge her to be "acting like a man," and violating gender norms. She is therefore seen as less likeable, making people less likely to vote for her. And when a woman does present herself in traditionally feminine ways, such as being nurturing, she is seen as not assertive and competent enough, and her chance of winning votes is also diminished.

The presidential campaigns of Hillary Clinton illustrate the difficulty of navigating this terrain. During her 2008 campaign for the Democratic party's nomination, for all intents and purposes, she ran "as a man." Her campaign focused on her experience, toughness, and considerable intelligence. She spoke often about foreign policy and less about "women's issues" like maternity leave. Her roles as a mother and daughter rarely came up and she avoided calling attention to her gender, as she did not want to be accused of playing a "gender card." And she lost. In retrospect, political analysts identify this as one of the major flaws of her campaign because it made her unrelatable and unlikeable.[32]

In her 2016 campaign, she changed tactics. Clinton often credited her role as a grandmother as a motivating factor in wanting to be president. She did not shy away from talking about the historic possibility of being the first female American president, discussed the empowerment of women broadly, and spoke personally of the sexist discrimination she has faced. At the same time, she worked to hold her ground on the "masculine" aspects of her candidacy: she and her surrogates continued to emphasize her intelligence and considerable experience.[33] And she lost again. We are still waiting for a female American president to break out of this ever-defeating conundrum.

## The Attractiveness Conundrum

Traditional gender roles also dictate the importance of attractiveness. A woman is doing femininity well if she is naturally attractive; if she isn't, she is expected to work at it through hairdos, makeup, clothes, and cosmetic surgeries. The worst insult my mother could say about a woman was that "she didn't take care of herself." People evaluate attractive women more positively than unattractive women, part of a phenomenon psychologists call "what is beautiful is good."[34] Under this spell, we tend to assume that physically attractive people are superior in many ways, including intelligence and overall personality. While my primary point here is about politics, it's worth first taking a look at how this plays out in dating and job interviewing.

Many studies show that, in general, attractive people are more popular and are considered to be more desirable dating partners than people not considered attractive. For men looking to date women, this preference is more pronounced than for women looking to date men.[35] Attractiveness also figures in to who gets hired for a job. An attractive man is more likely to be hired than an unattractive man in any type of job. For women, this works differently. An attractive woman is more likely to be hired for a job than an unattractive woman only if the job requires traditionally female qualities. If the job requires typically male qualities, an attractive woman is less likely to be hired.[36]

And in politics, the role of attractiveness is even more complicated. How people evaluate a candidate very much depends on the gender of the candidate. For men, attractiveness is not an issue as long as they are reasonably groomed, but a woman's perceived attractiveness works as a double-edged sword. In the 2008 presidential election, we saw this judgment play out both ways.[37] The media made a lot of fuss about Republican vice presidential candidate Sarah Palin's attractiveness—she was referred to as a "MILF" and pictures of her in a bathing suit were aired widely. Buttons calling Palin the "Hottest VP" were worn at the Republican National Convention. The McCain campaign thought her attractiveness would be an asset, but it quickly devolved into a liability when the press dubbed her "Caribou Barbie" and *Newsweek* ran a cover picture of her in running shorts[38] that even the candidate called sexist. After she was nominated, one of the most popular political Internet searches was "Sarah Palin naked." Certainly, Palin's performances in television interviews didn't help convey an impression of competence, but her sexualization further diminished her stature as a candidate. On the flip side, Hillary Clinton's perceived lack of sexuality and attractiveness was used as a bludgeon. Buttons that said "KFC Hillary Special: 2 fat thighs, 2 small breasts...left wing" were sold at 2016 Republican events.[39]

How many women—how many *people*—would want to expose themselves to this seemingly no-win criteria? When fewer women run for political office, fewer women gain political power, and the imbalance persists.

## IT'S THE MYTH ITSELF THAT TRAPS US

The hormone myth is a strand of biological essentialism. Building on this worldview that our sex chromosomes (which involve two of the forty-six chromosomes every human has) and our corresponding reproductive roles are the most basic facts about us, gender polarization (the belief that there are two genders and that they are in many ways opposites) and our basic need to generalize about our world (that is, to stereotype), combine to form the deep-seated beliefs that explain the tremendous staying power of the hormone myth. The social rewards to women and girls for conforming to sweet, soft, kind femininity are reliable; the punishments for being "shrill" or sharp-edged or dominant are quick and sure. It's therefore easy to see how these beliefs become internalized, and why we want to find some safe explanation for the times when we don't measure up. Even women whose personal reality is contrary to the hormone myth create ways to think of themselves as special or unusual, maintaining the belief in the hormonal irrationality of women as a whole.

Given the damage that maintaining the hormone myth does to women, and to men as well, dismantling it is essential to the well-being of women and girls, and of humans generally. Accepting it, going along with it, even perpetuating it is relatively easy: so many pillars of our economic and political systems benefit from it, and so many strands of culture and society reinforce it blindly.

If we find we are buying it, selling it, or using it against other women or ourselves, we need to step back and ask ourselves why. Is our rage or sadness or not-niceness so meaningless—or so dangerous—that it can only be released when there are hormones to blame, when we can be so easily ridiculed and dismissed? What true things are not being said? What parts of our selves—and of our daughters and sisters and mothers—are we denying? Is this really the way we want to be?

# Protecting the Powerful Reality of Women

Myths about gender have a lot of power. They are generated by a combination of cultural, social, and economic values, and enacted by major institutions like government, religion, and industry. They strongly influence our ideas of what men and women are like: that they should act and feel a certain way, and that it is inevitable that they do so. Myths dictate the roles we expect men and women to play and their storylines about the nature of women create a distinct disadvantage. The myths about women's psychological health, as it relates to reproductive processes, that I've examined and debunked in this book are particularly pernicious and resistant to change.

## THE GOOD NEWS

When we critically look at the errors in thinking and scientific methods applied to questions about women's reproductive and mental health, and reveal the motivations for maintaining these myths—which often have nothing to do with protecting women's health—women gain the freedom to reconceptualize the meaning of our reproductive processes in healthy, positive ways. Here is a review of the good news we now know about women.

## Menstruation Can Be Seen as Natural and Anger Can Be Expressible

Activists are working to change the perception of menstruation so that it's no longer a woman's private, shameful burden and is instead seen as a normal, biological process. Bold and innovative social movements are working to take the shame out of menstruation with the purpose of gaining "menstrual equity." Groups like Girls Helping Girls Period are working to make pads and tampons easily available through a general acknowledgement that these are necessities for menstruating girls and women. Bizarrely, up until 2015, most states taxed menstrual products as a luxury item. A luxury? I can't imagine any woman thinking of her pad or tampon as a special thing she gets just to feel good. A 2016 legislation sweep, which *New York* magazine described as "viral," introduced laws to abolish the tax in many states and New York City passed legislation to fund providing menstrual products in public schools, homeless shelters, and prisons.[1] This work is also important in places like Uganda, Kenya, and Nepal, where girls are often ostracized and made to stay home from school when they have their periods.[2] Equal access to education is one of the most powerful tools to minimize gender inequality and attitudes about menstruation have been a major obstacle to overcoming it.

It is important to acknowledge that there is a small percentage of women who experience disturbing *physical* symptoms from menstruation, and that hormones do play a role. At the same time, expectations of these negative physical symptoms do contribute to negative experiences. So while the widespread messages women receive about "menstrual misery" are not only false for most women, they contribute to some women's experience of menstruation as "the curse."

Given that, imagine for a moment what would happen if we completely reframed menstruation as a positive thing. Would our suffering decrease? It's fun to imagine that possibility. In Gloria Steinem's legendary essay, "If Men Could Menstruate," she playfully imagines the positive spin men would put on menstruating if they did: they would brag about it, have parties to celebrate it, and—simply because men did it—menstruation would lose its shameful and hidden status.[3] The essay was written tongue-in-cheek, but all the same, it points to a possible reality in which menstruation is a badge of honor rather than a stigma. What if it came to be seen as a reflection of the awesome power to create life that women have?

Just imagine how that would make us feel about our bodies, and ourselves. Perception powerfully shapes experience.

It is also true that a small percentage of women do experience disturbing *emotional* symptoms due to the menstrual cycle—which reflects a very specific condition now more appropriately identified as PMDD. But for most women, what's going on in our daily lives plays a more important role in predicting moods than changes in hormone levels.

Exposing the flimsy artifices that make up the myth of PMS makes it possible to reveal important truths about women's emotional health. By focusing on high-quality research and cutting through the massive campaign waged to convince women of the ubiquity of PMS, we can highlight important facts about the positive reality of women's mental health in relation to menstruation: time of the month and the concurrent changes in reproductive hormones do not adversely affect women's abilities to function, as neither intellectual skills, nor spatial skills, nor motor skills, nor memory, are affected; the great majority of women emotionally function at a high level across the month; monthly changes in hormone levels have no influence on most women's moods; women are generally no moodier than men. What we need to work on, as a culture, is allowing women to express their anger, to own it, and to appreciate what it points out about what's wrong in a situation. With all that in mind, I can confidently say: ditch the image of the PMSing bitch. It simply isn't true to life.

## Pregnant Women Can Function

The good news is that there is no consistent evidence that pregnant women lose their memory, verbal abilities, or ability to concentrate. The few studies that do find a negative impact of pregnancy find very small differences during specific weeks. And importantly, we know that the inevitable changes in hormones during pregnancy don't hurt women's abilities to think or be emotionally rational. Think about yourself or pregnant women you've known. It's likely that you functioned quite well in your everyday responsibilities while pregnant. Being pregnant isn't easy and sometimes some physical accommodations are reasonable to ask for. But there is no reason to think that pregnant women don't do what we women have always done—reliably taking care of the tasks of life. And the more this truth is publicized, the better the status of pregnant women will become.

## Postpartum Depression is Highly Preventable

Postpartum depression is real and is experienced by about 10 percent of women, but a convincing number of studies show that it is not caused by changes in hormones. The strongest indicator that a woman will suffer from postpartum depression is being depressed during pregnancy, so if doctors evaluated women and provided treatment while pregnant, they could greatly decrease the number of women who experience this disorder. Other factors that contribute include childcare stress and poor social support. This realization emphasizes the very gendered nature of caring for babies and how it threatens women's mental health. If more partners, husbands, family members, and social circles truly shared in childcare duties—beyond just "helping out" from time to time—and we got past the idea that one woman, in isolation, is the best way to care for an infant, mothering a new baby could become a less overwhelming task, and fewer women would suffer from depression at this time.

## Menopause Brings Women Choice and Freedom

Neither hormone levels, nor stage of menopause, are related to women's mental health. This leaves a much more optimistic picture to appreciate. Most women describe the changes that perimenopause and menopause bring as minor and manageable. Studies show that most women of menopausal age are not depressed and are indeed happy with their lives. Women can look forward to their fifties and sixties as a decades of rejuvenation and freedom. Free from periods, pregnancy, and the daily work of raising children, this stage of life comes with all kinds of possibilities to refocus priorities on our needs and desires.

Many women feel like their accumulated wisdom helps them to know who they are and who they want to be. This self-confidence also translates to trusting an inner voice and feeling comfortable using it. While in Western culture, getting older for women is associated with irrelevancy and inevitable decline, the good news is that for most women, this couldn't be further from the truth. You don't need to look far to find menopausal or postmenopausal women who are happy, energized, and highly productive. These women are all around us, and that is something to celebrate. The menopausal years bring a wonderful opportunity for women to aim high and live life on their terms.

# TOOLS YOU CAN USE TO DEFEND AGAINST THE HORMONE MYTH

Propagating the false assumptions of the hormone myth costs all of us way more than it's worth. Women are competent, rational, and highly functional people. Think about what you get done in a day! An emotionally erratic, mentally ill person could not achieve what you do. And it's not fair that despite all the daily evidence to the contrary, you can be cut down with the hormone myth. "It's just your hormones" is an unacceptable and invalidating insult. But it is in your power to resist and deflate this lie. Here are useful tools to combat it.

## Skepticism

Be skeptical of any assertions involving the hormone myth. You are now armed with an informed understanding of what drives the myth and how it has forged public consciousness. Foremost, be skeptical of the human need to categorize. Categorizing people is necessary to bring order to our brains, but it often happens based on limited or faulty information. To come to a more accurate perception of the relationship between women's reproductive functions and their mental health, try to defy easy categorizations. Evaluate people based on your interactions with them, rather than established categories, so you can more accurately see their natures and abilities.

Another trigger for alarm bells is anything that maintains traditional gender roles to effectively give men more power than women. When a woman's competency is questioned because of hormonal changes during menstruation, pregnancy, or menopause, the suspicions that the hormone myth perpetuates are validated—which makes keeping us out of powerful positions seem reasonable. Your skepticism can keep disempowerment from making sense.

Even medical practitioners, like physicians and psychologists, benefit financially from labeling women's reproductive processes as illnesses because doing so gives them more patients to "treat." So keep your healthy skepticism, especially when facing the illusion of impartiality and authority that doctors try to uphold, and listen for signs of the hormone myth at work.

Because you now know the hormone myth has provided the pharmaceutical companies with an endless gravy train worth billions of dollars in annual revenue—despite little evidence that "treatments" for PMS or menopause are necessary or useful—you can identify the hype for what it is. They have a lot of motivation to keep selling lies to American women, so it's critical for you to remember that none of the forces that propel the hormone myth are motivated by a sincere interest in promoting or protecting women's health.

Stay alert for bad science. I have filled this book with examples of it, and if you want to further arm yourself to identify it and sort good studies from flawed ones, do read appendix II: "Ways to Spot Junk Science." In chapter 3, I reviewed the stunning number of critical flaws in studies done up until the 1980s that supported the existence of a premenstrual syndrome, flaws that render the majority of the findings invalid. So before you accept something because "science" says so, examine the research behind it.

Be especially skeptical of the ways the media reports research results. Findings that support the fundamental idea supporting the hormone myth—that men and women are different—are much more likely to be published than studies that find no differences, so be aware that you generally hear only one version of reality. Popular news sources skew it even further because reporters truncate details and even report study findings inaccurately to fit a narrative they prefer. When scientific research is misrepresented so that it supports the hormone myth, it seeps into the public consciousness through websites, television shows, and books, which all present the accepted—but wrong—image of women at the mercy of their hormones.

Your awareness of the forces driving the hormone myth and how they implant it in the popular zeitgeist can take away their power to dictate your thoughts and feelings about women. Use it to foster a perception of women that is closer to reality.

## Honesty

A fundamental idea that perpetuates the hormone myth is that women should always be nice and pleasant. Belief in this standard makes the hormone myth very useful for women, as we can maintain our self-concept of being a good woman by attributing any anger to hormones. Feeling angry is uncomfortable for most women. I hope that I've opened you to the idea that, when you are feeling negative emotions like anger or sadness—while there is a small possibility that it is because of hormonal change—it is much more probable that something else is the cause. If you want to figure out what that might be, you need to be honest with yourself.

Naming what upsets us can be scary because then the ball is in our court. But we can't move forward in our lives and grow without doing so. It can be difficult to take a hard look at life and realize some things are not how we want them: one woman might hate the company culture at her job, and another might be exhausted from caring for a sick mother. But figuring out what is upsetting us puts us on the road to figuring out how to help ourselves feel better.

You can feel better because if you are honest, you can work to change your situation. And if you realize that, for now, your situation is not going to change, you can find more beneficial ways of coping with it. This process can begin as soon as you, personally, push the hormone myth aside.

Here's a sample scenario. You come home from work and the house is a wreck for the umpteenth time. Neither your kids nor husband have done any cleaning, even though you left them a to-do list. You show your anger by saying something like: "Would it be so hard to clean up the toys? Do I have to come home to a destroyed house every day?" From his place in front of the television, your husband says, "What's the matter with you, are you on the rag?" The menstruation accusation has been thrown. But you know your anger is justified—and that it has nothing to do with your time of the month. How to proceed from here?

Traditional ideas about dividing duties by gender don't have to dictate what we think we deserve—when the hormone myth is used to counter a woman's dissatisfaction, it represents an *avoidance* response. It's an attempt to change the focus from the situation at hand to a woman's supposedly irrational and uncontrollable body. Not only is this response demeaning to women, it's bad for a relationship. When couples avoid discussions about actions and feelings that cause conflict, this can cause chronic interpersonal tension and issues are never resolved.[4]

The ways in which we express dissatisfaction matter. Express your feelings and position by first stopping the menstruation accusation in its tracks, whether in the moment or in a separate conversation. Tell your husband, boyfriend, or partner how hurtful and invalidating it is for him to suggest that your anger is only because of hormones and not because of the reality of his actions. Then bring the conversation back to the issue at hand—his actions. Even humor might help: "That's so weird that you would bring up my period when what we're talking about is the way the house is always a mess when I come home."

Just as you can benefit tremendously by resisting default messages about hormones in your own life, countering the messages in other people's heads is equally powerful. Will you laugh at the menstruation jokes now? And when a woman shows anger and she's invalidated by the hormone accusation, either to her face or behind her back, how would you respond now that you're aware of what's actually happening? By being honest with yourself and with others, everyone will benefit because you are now addressing the reality of situations.

## Generosity

When a friend vehemently complains about something, and then apologizes by saying she is just "PMSing" or "all preggo" or "being menopausal," you can acknowledge that we've all gotten the hormone message loud and clear. But add that there is convincing research that most women's hormones don't affect their emotional state. You can gently suggest that she's allowed to be angry and doesn't need to apologize for it. Women have strongly internalized the hormone myth, and while it won't be easy to convince them otherwise, it is a worthwhile effort. Responding to their negative emotions with acceptance and engagement, rather than disapproval and dismissal, is a good start.

A powerful strategy for resisting the hormone myth is to promote a spirit of generosity when judging yourself and others. Men and women have moods that change from time to time, and this is completely normal. Women sometimes feel anger and men sometimes feel sadness. Emotions are caused by a wide array of situational factors, like happy occasions or stressful conditions, and for most people this has very little to do with reproductive hormones. Traditional gendered expectations about how women and men should feel—and should express those feelings—are restrictive and can be soul-crushing. Accepting and embracing the variety of the human condition can be liberating for everyone.

One caveat—it is important not to dismiss the *physical* problems that can be associated with women's reproductive functions. Painful cramps, polycystic ovary syndrome (PCOS), and endometriosis are all examples of well-documented biological disorders that some women experience, and hormonal changes do play a role. I am by no means suggesting that these disorders don't exist or require treatment. They should be taken seriously. Women who suffer from these physical disorders can experience strong emotional responses to these conditions and are deserving of sympathy, treatment, and acceptance.

## Taking Action

You can work to fight the hormone myth by speaking up when you hear it. These days, voices are loudly heard online, as on blogs, Facebook, and Twitter, both national and international discussions take place on the topics of the day. Collective voices rose up in 2016 when, after a presidential debate Donald Trump criticized journalist Megyn Kelly's aggressive questions with the period accusation. The Internet lit up as millions of people, with low and high profiles, rejected his reasoning as false and misogynistic. Many people are ready to dispute, and even walk away from, the hormone myth—and social media platforms can influentially project this message. That power is in your hands. So the next time you hear or read that women are hormonal maniacs, trust your truth and use your voice to deflate the hormone myth. Spread the good news that there is abundant research showing that hormones rarely affect women's mental health and that the great majority of women are high-functioning most of the time.

## RAISING BOYS AND GIRLS TO RESIST THE HORMONE MYTH

An even longer-lasting strategy you can use to contest the biological-essentialism assumption is to raise children to reject the idea that women are at the mercy of their hormones. Boys and girls often get their introduction to the hormone myth when they learn about menstruation. The preteen years is a great time to provide accurate information about women's bodies and women's emotions.

## Menstrual Attitudes for Girls

Probably because they actually experience menstruation and can become pregnant, more time and effort is put into educating girls about puberty and reproduction than boys.[5] Culturally, girls get mixed messages: they may learn that a monthly menstrual cycle is healthy and natural, and they also can't miss the shameful connotation menstrual blood has through the necessary efforts they must make to keep it hidden.[6]

Mothers have a unique opportunity to provide daughters with accurate information about menstruation. You may think that a preteen doesn't want to have "that conversation" with her mother, but it turns out she may want to have several conversations. One study of ten- and twelve-year-old girls found that they want *more* information and advice from their parents on the subjects of puberty and sexuality.[7] And college-aged women report that being educated by their mothers before menstruation started was very useful in reducing fears or anxieties about it.[8]

If you are a mother, take this opportunity to teach your girls the reassuring truth: that the physical changes of the menstrual cycle will not adversely affect their ability to cognitively function and that it is very unlikely that it will affect them emotionally to an extreme degree. It doesn't need to be one big conversation. Mothers can talk to their daughters matter-of-factly when they have their periods, so it is a normalized subject to begin with. You can convey information about the logistics of self-care—which is what most girls are concerned about—and take the shame out of menstruation simply by talking about it.

When girls run into the inevitable jokes and misinformation about PMS, you can teach your daughters to be critical of these messages about women. When a mother initiates these conversations about menstruation with her daughter, future conversations about sexuality and other sensitive topics become less of a big deal.[9]

## Teaching Boys About Women's Bodies

Since the focus of the hormone myth is on women's bodies as being different from men's and therefore impaired, it is important to teach girls accurate information and discourage the development of stereotypes. But in order to work toward ending the hormone myth and all its negative consequences, teaching boys accurate information is equally important. Men's sustained perceptions that women's psychological health is regularly threatened by reproductive processes are particularly influential because of the greater social, economic, and political power men hold.

Boys receive much less education about puberty than girls.[10] While there are concerted efforts from schools and mothers to educate girls about their bodies through classes and conversations, boys grab details where they can. In a rare study of how boys learn about menstruation, male college students reported first learning about it when one of their sisters began to menstruate. Without parents or schools offering organized information, many felt confused and ignorant, and had to sift through the often unreliable information provided by peers. The men in the study reported that a common theme they learned when young is: menstruation is disgusting and should be hidden. Several men remembered incidents when girls were severely teased if their menstruation was revealed.[11]

The men in the study who grew to develop more positive views reported that the most influential events were individual conversations they had with a girlfriend. Intimate, private conversations within a respectful frame made it possible for these men to gain a more accurate, and less misogynistic, view of menstruation. This speaks to the potential power mothers and fathers can have in helping boys to altogether skip the phase of ridiculing girls' bodies over something they fear and don't understand. A mother can model a positive attitude about the way her body works and how it doesn't impede her mental and physical abilities. She can make a point to buy tampons in front of her son, and fathers can model a respectful perspective.

Both mothers and fathers can teach their sons about the unfairness of stereotypes. If a son has a sister, they can say something like, "You wouldn't want someone trying to shame her or say what she can't do because she is a girl, would you?" And even better, they can turn it around and say, "You wouldn't want someone telling you something natural about your body is disgusting and that there are things you can't do because you're a boy."

# LEADING THE WAY TO POSITIVE, EMPOWERING IMAGES OF WOMEN

There is a lot of reason for optimism. Especially because, when people become aware of the faulty science and insidious agendas the hormone myth is based on, it becomes easy to walk away from. Young women are leading the way to a new conceptualization of gender and the body, as reproductive physiology no longer holds an important role in dictating their behavior and they view it more matter-of-factly. For these women, bodily issues surrounding periods, birth control, pregnancy, and sexuality are presented neutrally and without taboo or shame. Many millennial women reject old gender binaries and traditional gender roles. They think of gender as much more complicated than simply male and female—to them, it exists on a fluid continuum.[12] When they consider future work-family models, they hope for egalitarian relationships in which homemaking and income-generating responsibilities are shared.[13] Despite the ubiquitous power of the hormone myth, the tide is changing.

The truth is that menstruation, pregnancy, and menopause, in and of themselves, do not harm women's mental health in any meaningful way, and that postpartum depression can be prevented. Life is so rich, complicated, and dynamic: attitudes, expectations, social structures, and economic factors are by far more influential on women's moods than these biological processes. By embracing and promoting the truth, that reproductive hormones are not related to women's mental health in any significant way, we can hail the reality that is clear to see: in all ways, most of us function at very high levels throughout our lives. This is the powerful truth about women.

# Acknowledgments

When I started this project, I thought, "Wow, I'm going to write a book!" Since then, I've figured out that no one writes a book alone. There are many people to acknowledge who helped this book happen. Foremost, I would like to thank my first editor extraordinaire, Clancy Drake. From the beginning, she understood my vision and shaped it in meaningful ways; I could not have asked for an editor who is smarter or more passionate. Special thanks go to my second editor, Jennifer Holder, who with great insight and gusto helped me bring this book to its final form. At New Harbinger, I appreciate how Julie Bennett's enthusiasm leads the way, and all the hard work the fearless marketing team put into getting this book into readers' hands.

I certainly didn't wake up one day ready to write a book. I am so grateful to my mentor, Marci Lobel, who brought me into the world of health psychology and provided me with excellent training as a graduate student. She has been an enthusiastic supporter of all my professional pursuits, and a great friend and colleague. I'd also like to thank Sally Sternglanz, who helped me find my feminist voice. Her encouragement never wavered and she gave me the confidence to expand my professional goals. Many thanks to the team at WAGS, especially Mary Jo Bona, who was an excellent boss and colleague.

I would like to thank Nancy Franklin, who spearheads the TEDx talks, for her great feedback when preparing for "The Good News About PMS," which was the launching point for this book. I so appreciate Jill Kramer, who believed in my idea and brought my proposal forward, and also my digital publicist, Spencer Smith, who offered tremendous practical help getting me into cyberspace.

A big shout out goes to the members of the women's networking group, Moxxie. These incredibly smart and super-competent women—CEO Beth Meixner, Dawn Davidson-Drantch, Grace Barry, Lisa Pomeranz, Dona Rutowicz, and many others—have given me generous personal and practical support for writing this book and developing my business. Special thanks to publicist Cecilia Alers for teaching me about branding and helping me wade into the world of social media. And to my accountability partner Joan Siegelwax Axelrod, a million thank-yous for keeping me on track, being a great friend, and giving the best advice ever.

Eternal thanks to my parents, Stan Stein and the late Barbara Stein, for raising me with such love and giving me the guts to try something like this. To my wonderful big sister, Kelly McAdam, how can I ever thank you enough for all the love and encouragement you give me? You are my best friend and I can't imagine my life without you. And to my dear brother, Brian Steinberg, truly a lifelong friend, thank you for the confidence you have in me and for being the first to order the book. To my daughters, Caroline and Jamie, you are both sweet, thoughtful people whose endless enthusiasm for my work means so much to me; thank you for enduring my endless babbling about the book in the last two years. Caroline, thank you for believing in me, for the incredibly useful editing advice you gave when this book was in its early stages, and for being patient with my annoying use of passive voice. Jamie, thank you for being my personal cheerleader, for jumping up and down with me when I was offered the contract, and for publicizing my TEDx talk on your Facebook page with the post "My mom is cooler than your mom." And to my new son-in-law, Gilad, many thanks for your thoughtful support, interest in this project, and your excellent marketing ideas.

And most importantly, a heartfelt thank you to Tony DeLuca for having supported any professional pursuit I set my mind to from the very beginning. Some husbands might mind if five minutes after the wedding, their wife said, "I'd like to quit my job and get a PhD," but not you. You believed in me and always did everything you could to help make my dreams come true. For that and so much more, I'm forever grateful.

**The Hormone Myth**

# Women's Hormones:
# An Overview

The word "hormones" gets thrown around a lot in conversations about women's health, but what exactly are they? In general, hormones are chemicals produced by the body that send messages to organs to help regulate biological processes. For example, adrenaline is a hormone produced by the adrenal glands that, among other things, makes your heart beat faster to facilitate action in response to a threat. It gets that old "flight or fight" response going. But when people talk about women and hormones, they usually are referring to *reproductive* hormones that work to regulate reproductive functioning like menstruation, pregnancy, and menopause. The primary female reproductive hormones are follicle stimulating hormone (FSH), luteinizing hormone (LH), estrogen, progesterone, and human chorionic gonadotropin (HCG). Here's a brief primer on how they work.[1]

### Follicle Stimulating Hormone (FSH)
FSH is secreted by the pituitary gland in the brain. Each month, it stimulates the growth of a follicle that produces an egg in the ovary.

### Luteinizing Hormone (LH)
LH is also secreted by the pituitary gland. It plays a part in the menstrual cycle by causing the production of estrogen in the ovary, and the release of the mature egg from the follicle.

### Estrogen
Estrogen is produced by several parts of the body: the ovaries, the adrenal glands, fatty tissue, and the placenta during pregnancy. In puberty, it

regulates the development of secondary sex characteristics like breasts and pubic hair. In menstruation, estrogen facilitates the growth of the uterine lining. Estrogen helps to maintain the lining during pregnancy, and plays an important role in the development of the fetus.

### Progesterone

Progesterone is secreted by the empty follicle that released the egg. It also helps to build up the lining of the uterus. In the first trimester of pregnancy, this hormone rises dramatically. It keeps the muscles of the uterus relaxed, and is instrumental in keeping the mother's immune system from rejecting the foreign DNA, also known as: the baby.

### Human Chorionic Gonadotropin (HCG)

HCG is the critical hormone produced during pregnancy. It is made by what eventually becomes the placenta and it stops monthly egg production. It also helps to increase levels of estrogen and progesterone in the first ten weeks of pregnancy. At-home pregnancy tests work by detecting the presence of this hormone.

During the month, if no implantation of an egg occurs, the higher levels of progesterone and estrogen cause a decrease in the production of LH and FSH, which in turn decrease progesterone and estrogen. This makes the blood vessels in the uterus constrict, decreasing the supply of nutrients to the lining. Prostaglandins, which are chemicals made by the uterine lining, cause the uterus to contract (here come the cramps!) and the lining is shed in the menstrual flow. In the years leading up to menopause, the levels of estrogen and progesterone start to fluctuate more dramatically during the monthly cycle, and then start to gradually decline, eventually becoming too low to maintain the menstrual cycle.[2]

# Ways to Spot Junk Science

There has been a cultural shift in the way people think about their health. Previously, great trust was placed in doctors and we believed they knew what was best for us. But during the cultural revolutions of the 1960s and 70s, when all kinds of authority were being questioned, scrutiny was also applied to health care. We are now encouraged to be knowledgeable about our medical conditions and to participate in decisions about treatment. One way we can do that is to learn about recent scientific research. But most of us don't read medical or psychology journals; instead, we rely on getting information about various findings from media news outlets. So we don't have access to long, detailed descriptions of studies—we get bite-sized tidbits through a short paragraph in a newspaper, thirty seconds on television news, or one paragraph on a website. Very few details can be provided. But when it comes to assessing whether a study is valid and reliable—meaning that you can count on its results to be accurate—details matter. When media outlets provide little information about a study, how can the average person know if it's junk science or good science? Try asking the following questions.

## PONDER: WHY IS THIS SENSATIONAL ENOUGH TO COVER?

Studies most likely to get media attention are those finding differences. For example, a study finding gender differences in parenting styles is much more likely to get attention with a headline like "Dads would rather play than scold!" than a study finding no differences. The selections often portray popular cultural beliefs that people like to hear confirmed. This is a bias in coverage of all scientific research. Despite the fact that finding no differences is as meaningful as finding differences, journal editors and the popular press don't see it that way—and the consumer ends up with incomplete information.

## CONSIDER: WHAT'S THE INFORMATION SOURCE?

When I was pregnant, I asked my obstetrician if it was still okay for me to use artificial sweeteners. She responded by giving me a pamphlet published by the manufacturers of the sweetener Equal—not the most neutral party to rely on for information. Many institutions benefit from publishing studies, including scientists, journals, media outlets, and pharmaceutical companies, and their priorities are sadly not always scientific validity and improved public health. So to be a careful consumer of research, begin by assuming that these parties have their best interests at heart—not yours. Then figure out which parties stand to gain from a particular study's results.

## ASK: WHO WAS STUDIED?

Who were the subjects of the study? Are they like you? Most psychology research is done with college students. About half of all Americans attend some college, which means half don't. The fact that those who don't are rarely studied suggests that the results found in these studies may only be relevant to those who attend college. Demographically speaking, they are a fairly limited group—mostly white and middle- to upper-class. A similar problem can be found in medical studies. Up until the 1990s, most medical studies were performed with only men, severely limiting the application of study results.[1] For decades, physicians thought the classic symptom of a heart attack was severe pain in the arm or a crushing pain in the chest. It turns out that those are only classic symptoms of a heart attack in *men*. Women having a heart attack tend to have much more diffuse symptoms, like nausea, shortness of breath, and back pain.[2] Leaving women out of medical research compromised their ability to be accurately diagnosed and get timely treatment.

# QUESTION: DID THIS STUDY ACTUALLY MEASURE WHAT YOU THINK IT DID?

A hypothesis is the question researchers are asking, such as "Are women in an unhappy marriage more likely to develop postpartum depression?" From the hypothesis, it's clear that the study is going to somehow measure the variables of women's marital satisfaction and postpartum depression. When you hear a result, compare it to the study's hypothesis to confirm that this was indeed what was being measured—rather than part of an introduction, a historical pattern, or a suggestion for further study. Authors of studies usually first discuss the results of previous studies on the topic and propose possible reasons for them—before describing the study they did. Make sure that the result you hear in the press reflects the actual study done, not a previous study or a simple speculation. The media mixes this up way too often.

Also look into whether standardized measures were used. These are tests that have been developed to measure a specific variable and have been tested previously to verify that it does indeed measure what researchers think it does. Let's go back to the sample hypothesis. Postpartum depression has been measured in a variety of ways, but one standardized measure commonly used is the Edinburgh Postnatal Depression Scale (EPDS). It is a list of ten statements like "In the past seven days, I've been anxious or worried for no good reason." A woman has the choice of rating each statement with "No, not at all," "Hardly ever," "Yes, sometimes," and "Yes, very often." These answers have numerical values, and are then totaled to create a score. Through extensive testing, the authors of this test established cutoff scores to identify women with depressed mood, and those without.[3] Asking a woman ten questions that focus on symptoms of depression provides an indication of her mood based on the multiple symptoms that may occur. Also, giving her options to rate the severity of each symptom gives a more detailed picture of her condition, and makes it possible to do detailed statistical analyses. What is good about a standardized measure is that when many different psychologists measure the same variable, like postpartum mood, a standardized measure allows them to do so in the exact same way, and therefore, studies can be confidently compared. Reviewers know the studies are comparing women with the same condition.

An unstandardized test is a methodologically weaker way to find out if women are depressed. It might simply ask women, "Are you depressed?"

The problem with this approach is that women can interpret this one question differently. Some may think being depressed means crying all the time, whereas others might think being depressed involves just having sad thoughts. There's no way to know.

## WONDER: WERE GOOD METHODS APPLIED?

The procedures used to test the hypothesis are called "the methods" of the study. These can get pretty complicated, but there are some basic conditions that substantially add to quality of a study.

### Were the Participants Randomly Assigned?

"Random assignment" refers to the procedure that begins with the group of study volunteers. Some individuals are randomly chosen to receive the experimental intervention, and some are randomly chosen to be part of the group that doesn't receive the experimental intervention. Randomly picking people to participate in a particular experimental group ensures that, overall, the people in each group are similar and that differences detected between the groups were due to the variable being tested—not something about the people who chose to be in a certain group.

For example, in the 1970s researchers carried out many experiments examining the influence of violent television shows on behavior in children.[4] The average study went something like this: each child was randomly assigned to either a group that watched a violent children's show or a group that watched a nonviolent show. Then they played with other children and any incidents of physical violence were documented. If the researchers had allowed the children to pick which show they wanted to watch, children who had more aggressive personalities might have been more likely to choose the violent show. Then, if they did tend to show more violent behavior afterwards, we wouldn't know if that was due to the variable of watching violent television, or the more aggressive personalities of the children in that group.

### Was There a Control Group?

A second important feature of reliable experiments is a "control group." A control group includes participants who ideally experience everything the same as the experimental group, except the variable being tested. In the study I described in the last section, almost everything these kids did was the same—they came to the lab, watched television, and played with children afterward. The only difference was in the content of the television show they watched. This creates the perfect comparison group. Researchers were able to compare the number of violent acts performed by the children who watched violent television to the number of violent acts performed by the children who watched nonviolent television, and have confidence that any differences found were due to the experimental variable of violent content.

## Where Were the Experiments Conducted?

It's also useful to know if the hypothesis is tested in a laboratory setting rather than a real-life situation. Much can be learned from lab studies, but they do raise questions about how well the findings from the study can be applied to real life. In the studies where children watched television in a lab, strong evidence was found that children who had watched the violent show were much more likely to hit or push other children in the time immediately following.

So should we believe that watching violent shows causes children to be physically violent? Not exactly. The experiments did a good job isolating the influence of violent television content as the cause of the violent behavior. But was it like watching television at home? Not really. When a child watches at home, his mother may stop to ask him questions, a sister may jump on him, or he may be distracted by a toy for much of the time. The undiluted dose of violent content given in the lab is not what children watching in real life get. So it wouldn't be appropriate to conclude that allowing children to watch violent television causes them to be physically violent. We can only conclude that it does—in some conditions.

## CHECK: WHO PAID FOR THE STUDY?

Research isn't cheap. Conducting studies requires staff to carry out the study, do the analyses, write it up, and submit the study for publication. Other costs include equipment and recruiting—and sometimes paying—participants. Long-term studies and those measuring biological markers can be especially costly, requiring budgets in the millions. Very few groups have that kind of money. A large percentage of medical and psychological studies conducted by researchers at colleges and universities in the United States are funded by grants from government agencies like the National Institutes of Health (NIH) or the Department of Health and Human Services (HHS). These allow maximum neutrality for the researchers, since the agencies are nonprofit and aren't going to produce a profit based on findings.

Studies funded by profit-oriented industries however, are another story. A pharmaceutical company's first commitment is to make money for stockholders. Not to improve public health. Not to cure disease. Profit maximization is the most important goal. The way they do this is by developing drugs and treatments that will be prescribed for large quantities of people for a long time. So when a pharmaceutical company funds a study, their financial interest in the outcome is paramount. These studies may be carried out by company scientists or by university researchers. In either case, when considering their outcome it's crucial to critically evaluate the methods of these studies. Did the drug or treatment outperform a placebo? Was the effect replicated in several trials? While studies funded by an industry financially invested in the outcome can be valid, the bar for the quality of the study methods needs to be set even higher.

## INVESTIGATE: WHAT HIDDEN AGENDAS ARE BEING PROMOTED?

When trying to figure out what is true and what is myth, it's important to understand what agendas may be at work. When it comes to women's health, there are many interested parties. Professional organizations like the American Psychological Association (APA), and the American Medical Association (AMA) are highly invested in the establishment of illnesses they can diagnose and treat. If they legitimize a disorder, then insurance companies will reimburse them for treatment. It's especially advantageous to give credibility to a disorder like PMS, which is supposed to afflict large numbers of women on a monthly basis for all of their childbearing years. Recent years have brought us official diagnoses for restless leg syndrome and social anxiety disorder—conditions previously thought of as within the normal range of the human condition. Yes, some people

**The Hormone Myth**

may find relief from debilitating conditions, but by making them official disorders the door opens to more income from doctor visits and prescription medication.

Ideological groups also have a stake in putting out information that supports their convictions. For example, pro-life groups have publicized the idea that abortion causes long-term psychological trauma, oftentimes through personal accounts of individual women. However, methodologically strong studies show no long-term trauma for most women having abortions.[5] On the other hand, some pro-choice groups suggest there are *no* psychological risks in having an abortion, which is not exactly true either. Studies show that there is a minority of women—about 15 percent—who do suffer long-term guilt and sadness after an abortion. It was found that these women frequently attended church, or struggled with the decision to have the abortion, or had initially wanted the pregnancy.[6] So while it's reasonable to think that people will have different opinions about the morality of abortion, we must be skeptical about information put forth in support of those opinions. As has been said many times: you get to have your own opinions, but you don't get to have your own facts.

## WATCH OUT: SOME RED FLAGS

Sometimes when a "fact" has been around for so long, it becomes socially and culturally entrenched, and people simply believe it's true. When we've heard something over and over again, it becomes part of our way of understanding the world. But just because everyone thinks something is true doesn't make it true. How can we navigate this? Here are a some red flags to get your radar up when considering the truth of something "everybody knows."

### When There Are Huge Profits Involved

If a particular accepted fact facilitates the accumulation of billions of dollars, or supports an industry, that should raise suspicion. Think about the herbal supplement ginko biloba. It is widely thought to improve memory and can be found in any vitamin aisle, can be added to smoothies, and is sold in herbal tea. However, several well-done studies have shown that it has very little, if any, effect on memory.[7] But that hasn't stopped herbal companies from publicizing its effectiveness, thereby maintaining highly profitable sales.

## When One Group Is Privileged Over Another

When a common belief suggests that some human beings are superior and therefore justified in their higher status, that's a good sign to become suspicious. This kind of belief is more likely to reflect a desire for power rather than a concerted effort to find the truth. One piece of received wisdom that has survived the ages is the idea that women are inferior to men, particularly intellectually. For centuries, women's inferior status was explained as being due to their female reproductive organs and their lack of male physiology. This sentiment was supported by biblical evidence (Eve caused the fall of man), and then philosophical reasoning (by Aristotle, Rousseau, and others). With the dawn of the scientific age, studies of the brain took up the mantle of female inferiority, although it took some major gymnastics to make the data fit the theory. In the 1850s, scientists began studying the brain, and concluded that the frontal lobes were responsible for intellectual activities. Almost immediately, several studies were published finding that male frontal lobes were much bigger than female frontal lobes, and female parietal lobes were larger than male parietal lobes. By the late in the century, however, there was a shift in thinking and it was decided that the part of the brain most responsible for intellect was the parietal lobe. Just as quickly, scientists revised their conclusions and reported that males had larger parietal lobes than women.[8] The belief that men are intellectually superior to women has been used to justify male dominance in most spheres of life, and every generation's authorities have manipulated the methods of the day to support that myth. When something "everyone knows" creates institutionalized privilege for one group over another, it warrants a heavy dose of suspicion.

## When One Study Makes It So

"New study proves eating blueberries prevents cancer!" Feverish headlines like this offer a good reason to step back and hold the champagne—no matter how well the research was done. One study cannot, on its own, provide proof of anything. There is always a statistical possibility that the results were found because of chance, not because of any actual relationship between the variables being tested. This possibility becomes smaller and smaller every time the experiment is replicated and the same results are found. Other confounding variables, like experimenter bias, may also create a false positive result. Therefore, to have confidence in the results of a study, a hypothesis needs to be tested several times, by several scientists.

## When Results from One Group Are Applied to Another

Biological research is often first done on animals before testing hypotheses on humans. This is for ethical and safety issues, but also because the life spans of animals, like mice, are much shorter than the human life span, so the effect of changes on longevity can be tested much more quickly. However, evidence found in animal studies shouldn't be immediately applied to human physiology because, although there are some biological similarities, there are substantial and meaningful differences that make this application premature. When you hear of a fantastic new discovery that has only been tested on rats, it's important to know that answering the next question—whether that discovery applies to humans—will take many more years of research, and that no matter how promising the treatment seemed, the answer may ultimately be no.

One example of jumping the gun on animal research involves caloric restriction and longevity. "Caloric restriction" refers to restricting the intake of food by 25 to 40 percent. In animal studies, caloric restriction is associated with longer life for fish, mice, cows, and dogs.[9] In a study of nonhuman primates, caloric restriction caused weight loss and lower triglycerides, but lifespan was not changed.[10] In the only randomized trial of humans, caloric restriction was related to weight loss, better blood pressure, and a decrease in overall cholesterol—however, it was only a two-year study, so the effect of caloric restriction on human longevity is still unknown. Despite that lack of evidence, many people jumped on the bandwagon and practice a "starvation diet" for longevity.[11] As anyone who doesn't have enough food can tell you, constant hunger can be a stressful, disturbing state. Those who follow this diet do so because they believe that it is worth the pain to live a longer life. But there is currently no evidence that, for humans, this is the case.

# BE AN EDUCATED CONSUMER OF RESEARCH

By understanding what goes into making a study reliable, and the many forces that can threaten reliability, you become an educated consumer of research. You will no longer be at the whim of the latest study, or of what the press decides is a newsworthy study to feature. Having a basic knowledge of how research is done gives you the tools to critically analyze the studies covered by the press. You become empowered to make health and lifestyle decisions based on well-established evidence, rather than the latest fad.

# Notes

## Introduction: The Myth That Traps Us

1. N. D. Smith, "Aristotle's Theory of Natural Slavery," *Phoenix* 37, no. 2 (1983): 109. doi:10.2307/1087451.

2. Thomas, *The Summa theologica of St. Thomas Aquinas* (London: Burns Oates & Washbourne, 1912).

3. H. Institoris, J. Sprenger, and C. S. Mackay, *Malleus Maleficarum* (Cambridge, UK: Cambridge University Press, 2006).

4. R. P. Maines, *The Technology of the Orgasm: "Hysteria," the Vibrator, and Women's Sexual Satisfaction* (Baltimore: Johns Hopkins University Press, 1999).

5. S. West and P. Dranov, *The Hysterectomy Hoax: A Leading Surgeon Explains Why 90% of All Hysterectomies Are Unnecessary and Describes All the Treatment Options Available to Every Woman, No Matter What Age* (New York: Doubleday, 1994).

## Chapter 1: Meet the Menstrual Monster and the PMSing Bitch

1. See http://www.always.com/en-us/tips-and-advice/your-first-period.

2. See http://www.pbskids.org and http://www.girlshealth.gov.

3. C. Natterson, *The Care and Keeping of You 2: The Body Book for Older Girls* (Wisconsin, MO: American Girl, 2013).

4. A. E. Figert, "Premenstrual Syndrome as Scientific and Cultural Artifact," *Integrative Physiological & Behavioral Science* 40, no. 2 (2005): 102–13. doi:10.1007/bf02734245.

5. J. C. Chrisler, J. G. Rose, S. E. Dutch, K. G. Sklarsky, and M. C. Grant, "The PMS Illusion: Social Cognition Maintains Social Construction," *Sex Roles* 54, no. 5–6 (2006): 371–76. doi:10.1007/s11199–006–9005–3.

6. N. J. Cobb, "The Biological and Physical Changes of Adolescence," *Adolescence* (Sunderland, MA: Sinauer Associates, 2010).

7. M. L. Marván, M. Islas, L. Vela, J. C. Chrisler, and E. A. Warren, "Stereotypes of Women in Different Stages of Their Reproductive Life: Data From Mexico and the United States," *Health Care for Women International* 29, no. 7 (2008): 673–87. doi:10.1080/07399330802188982.

8.  T. Roberts, J. L. Goldenberg, C. Power, and T. Pyszczynski, "'Feminine Protection': The Effects of Menstruation on Attitudes Towards Women," *Psychology of Women Quarterly* 26, no. 2 (2002): 131–139.

9.  T. E. Jackson, and R. J. Falmagne, "Women Wearing White: Discourses of Menstruation and the Experience of Menarche," *Feminism & Psychology* 23, no. 3 (2013): 379–98. doi:10.1177/0959353512473812.

10. I. Johnston-Robledo and J. C. Chrisler, "The Menstrual Mark: Menstruation as Social Stigma," *Sex Roles* 68, no. 1–2 (2011): 9–18. doi:10.1007/s11199–011–0052-z.

11. L. Rosewarne, "The Menstrual Mess: The Disgust, Horror, and Fear of Menstruation," *Periods in Pop Culture* (United Kingdom: Lexington Books, 2012).

12. J. C. Chrisler et al., "The PMS Illusion."

13. L. Rosewarne, "The Menstrual Mess."

14. M. W. Matlin, "From Menarche to Menopause: Misconceptions about Women's Reproductive Lives," *Psychology Science* 45 (2003):106–22; B. Sommer, "Cognitive Performance and the Menstrual Cycle," *Cognition and the Menstrual Cycle*, ed. J. T. E. Richardson (New York, NY: Springer-Verlag, 1992).

15. I. S. Poromaa, and M. Gingnell, "Menstrual Cycle Influence on Cognitive Function and Emotion Processing—from a Reproductive Perspective," *Frontiers in Neuroscience* 8 (2014). doi:10.3389/fnins.2014.00380.

16. M. Gurevich, "Rethinking the Label," *Women & Health* 23, no. 2 (1995): 67–98. doi:10.1300/j013v23n02_05.

17. M. L. Stubbs, and D. Costos, "Negative Attitudes Toward Menstruation," *Women & Therapy* 27, no. 3–4 (2004): 37–54. doi:10.1300/j015v27n03_04.

18. A. M. Houston, A. Abraham, Z. Huang, and L. J. D'Angelo, "Knowledge, Attitudes, and Consequences of Menstrual Health in Urban Adolescent Females," *Journal of Pediatric and Adolescent Gynecology* 19, no. 4 (2006): 271–75. doi:10.1016/j.jpag.2006.05.002.

19. A. J. Barsky, "Nonspecific Medication Side Effects and the Nocebo Phenomenon," *JAMA* 287, no. 5 (2002): 622. doi:10.1001/jama.287.5.622.

20. M. G. Myers, J. A. Cairns, and J. Singer, "The Consent Form as a Possible Cause of Side Effects," *Clinical Pharmacology and Therapeutics* 42, no. 3 (1987): 250–53. doi: 10.1038/clpt.1987.142.

21. H. Leventhal, D. R. Nerenz, and A. Strauss, "Self-regulation and the Mechanisms for Symptom Appraisal." *Monograph Series in Psychosocial Epidemiology 3: Symptoms, Illness Behavior, and Help-seeking*, ed. D. Mechanic, 55–86. (New York: Neale Watson, 1982).

22. P.K. Klebanov and J. B. Jemmott, "Effects of Expectations and Bodily Sensations on Self-Reports of Premenstrual Symptoms," *Psychology of Women Quarterly* 16, no. 3 (1992): 289–310. doi:10.1111/j.1471–6402.1992.tb00256.x; C. Mcfarland, Michael Ross, and Nancy Decourville, "Women's Theories of Menstruation and Biases in Recall of Menstrual Symptoms." *Journal of Personality and Social Psychology* 57, no. 3 (1989): 522–31. doi:10.1037//0022–3514.57.3.522; S. T. Sigmon, K. J. Rohan, N. E. Boulard, D. M. Dorhofer, and S. R. Whitcomb. "Menstrual Reactivity: The Role of Gender-specificity, Anxiety, Sensitivity, and Somatic Concerns in Self-Reported Menstrual Distress." *Sex Roles* 43 (2000): 143–61.

23. I. Johnston-Robledo et al., "The Menstrual Mark," 9–18.

24. Ibid.; T. Roberts, "Female Trouble: The Menstrual Self-Evaluation Scale and Women's Self-Objectification." *Psychology of Women Quarterly* 28, no. 1 (2004): 22–26. doi: 10.1111/j.1471–6402.2004.00119.x.

25. M. E. Mcpherson and Lauren Korfine, "Menstruation Across Time: Menarche, Menstrual Attitudes, Experiences, and Behaviors." *Women's Health Issues* 14, no. 6 (2004): 193–200. doi:10.1016/j.whi.2004.08.006.

26. J. K. Rempel and B. Baumgartner, "The Relationship Between Attitudes Toward Menstruation and Sexual Attitudes, Desires, and Behavior in Women." *Archives of Sexual Behavior* 32 (2014): 155–63.

27. D. Schooler, L. M. Ward, A. Merriwether, and A. S. Caruthers, "Cycles of Shame: Menstrual Shame, Body Shame, and Sexual Decision-Making," *Journal of Sex Research* 42, no. 4 (2005): 324–334.

28. Z. Valentine, "The Percentage of Female CEOs in the Fortune 500 Drops to 4%," *Fortune*, June 16, 2016, http://fortune.com/2016/06/06/women-ceos-fortune-500-2016/.

29. K. Thompson, "Women's Groups Target Sexism in Campaigns," *Washington Post*, September 2, 2010, http://www.washingtonpost.com/wp-dyn/content/article/2010/09/01/AR2010090106849.html.

30. A. Phillips, "Donald Trump Keeps Bullying Megyn Kelly on Twitter Because Donald Trump." *Washington Post*, August 25, 2015, https://www.washingtonpost.com/news/the-fix/wp/2015/08/25/donald-trump-keeps-bullying-megyn-kelly-on-twitter-because-donald-trump/.

31. E. Yuko, "How the Period Paradox Keeps Women Down." *Ms. Magazine*, February 24, 2016, http://msmagazine.com/blog/2016/02/24/how-the-period-paradox-keeps-women-down/; E. Whelan, "A Patronizing 'Period Policy' Should Make Women's Blood Boil." *International Business Times*, March 3, 2016.

32. N. Bakalar, "PMS Symptoms Linked to Diet." *New York Times*, March 4, 2013; A. Waldman, "All the Rage." *New York Times*, February 15, 2012.

33. L. Johannes, "Does Calcium Lessen the Symptoms of PMS?" *Wall Street Journal*, December 16, 2008; "Stress Can Make PMS Symptoms Worse—Study." *Wall Street Journal*. August 23 2010.

34. D. Heller, "Why PMS Should Be Taken Seriously," Dr.Oz.com. June 21, 2012, accessed January 10, 2016, http://www.doctoroz.com/blog/daniel-heller-nd/why-pms-should-be-taken-seriously.

35. "PMS Health Center," WebMD, accessed July 20, 2016, http://www.webmd.com/women/pms/default.htm.

36. M. Pick, "PMS—A Preview of Perimenopause." *Woman to Woman*, accessed July 5, 2016, https://www.womentowomen.com/pms/pms-a-preview-of-perimenopause/.

37. R. Schultze, *Shape*, "The Best Way to Reduce Your PMS Symptoms, According to Science," July 7, 2016; S. Weiss, *Glamour*, "What to Eat to Make Your Period Suck Less," June 20, 2016; Z. Barnes, *Self*, "8 Habits that are Making Your Period Even Worse," August 1, 2016; L. Leonardi, *Good Housekeeping*, "7 Natural Period Remedies that Actually Work," January 21, 2016; L. Beck, *Cosmopolitan*, "9 SUPERReal Period Things All Dudes Need to Understand," May 22 2016.

38. C. Lorre, "The Good Guy Fluctuation." *The Big Bang Theory*, CBS, aired October 27, 2011.

39. E. Meriwether, "Menzies," *The New Girl*, FOX, aired November 13, 2012.

40. "PMS Jokes," *Pinterest*, accessed July 15, 2016, https://www.pinterest.com/explore/pms -jokes/.

41. L.J. Thornton, "'Time of the Month' on Twitter: Taboo, Stereotype and Bonding in a No-Holds-Barred Public Arena," *Sex Roles* 68, no. 1–2 (2011): 41–54. doi:10.1007/s 11199–011–0041–2.

42. M. E. Heilman, "Description and Prescription: How Gender Stereotypes Prevent Women's Ascent Up the Organizational Ladder," *Journal of Social Issues* 57, no. 4 (2001): 657–74. doi:10.1111/0022–4537.00234.

43. J. D'Emilio, "Battered Woman Syndrome and Premenstrual Syndrome: A Comparison of Their Possible Use as Defenses to Criminal Liability." *St: John's Law Review* 59, no, 3 (1985):558–57.

44. B. L. Jacobs, "PMS HAHAcronym: Perpetuating Male Superiority." *Texas Journal of Women and the Law* 14 (2004): 1–26.

45. *Rottenecards.com*, accessed January 28, 2016.

46. S. Hensley, "California Milk Board Dumps Controversial PMS Campaign," *NPR.org*, July 22, 2011, http://www.npr.org/sections/health-shots/2011/07/22/138600837/calif -milk-board-dumps-controversial-pms-campaign.

47. M. E. Heilman, "Description and Prescription."

48. N. J. Cobb, "The Biological and Physical Changes of Adolescence."

49. J. Lee, "'A Kotex and a Smile': Mothers and Daughters at Menarche," *Journal of Family Issues* 29, no. 10 (2008): 1325–347. doi:10.1177/0192513x08316117.

50. M. E. McPherson and L. Korfine, "Menstruation across Time: Menarche, Menstrual Attitudes, Experiences, and Behaviors," *Women's Health Issues* 14, no. 6 (2004): 193– 200. doi:10.1016/j.whi.2004.08.006.

51. E. J. Susman and L. D. Dorn. "Puberty: Its Role in Development." *Handbook of Adolescent Psychology*, ed. R. M. Lerner and L. Steinberg (Hoboken: John Wiley and Sons, 2009).

52. Ibid; N. J. Cobb, "The Biological and Physical Changes of Adolescence."

53. T. Hollenstein and J. P. Lougheed, "Beyond Storm and Stress: Typicality, Transactions, Timing, and Temperament to Account for Adolescent Change," *American Psychologist* 68, no. 6 (2013): 444–54. doi:10.1037/a0033586.

54. N. J. Cobb, "The Biological and Physical Changes of Adolescence."

55. R. Larson and M. H. Richards, *Divergent Realities: The Emotional Lives of Mothers, Fathers, and Adolescents* (New York: BasicBooks, 1994).

56. L. M. Derose, M. P. Shiyko, H. Foster, and J. Brooks-Gunn. "Associations Between Menarcheal Timing and Behavioral Developmental Trajectories for Girls from Age 6 to Age 15." *Journal of Youth and Adolescence* 40, no. 10 (2011): 1329–342. doi:10.1007/s 10964–010–9625–3.

57. A. Caspi and T. E. Moffitt, "Individual Differences Are Accentuated during Periods of Social Change: The Sample Case of Girls at Puberty," *Journal of Personality and Social Psychology* 61, no. 1 (1991): 157–68. doi:10.1037//0022–3514.61.1.157.

58. N. J. Cobb, "The Biological and Physical Changes of Adolescence."

# Chapter 2: Only Flawed Research and Profit Back PMS

1. For reviews see I. S. Poromaa et al., "Menstrual Cycle Influence on Cognitive Function and Emotion Processing—from a Reproductive Perspective"; B. Sommer "Cognitive Performance and the Menstrual Cycle."

2. R. T. Frank, "The Hormonal Causes of Premenstrual Tension," *Archives of Neurology and Psychiatry* 26, no. 5 (1931): 1053. doi:10.1001/archneurpsyc.1931.02230110151009.

3. A. E. Figert, *Women and the Ownership of PMS: The Structuring of a Psychiatric Disorder* (New York: Aldine De Gruyter, 1996).

4. R. Greene and K. Dalton. "The Premenstrual Syndrome," *British Medical Journal* 1 (1953): 1007–014.

5. K. Dalton, "Effect of Menstruation on Schoolgirls' Weekly Work," *British Medical Journal* 1, no. 5169 (1960): 326–28. doi:10.1136/bmj.1.5169.326.

6. M. B. Parlee, "The Premenstrual Syndrome," *Psychological Bulletin* 80 (1973): 454–65.

7. J. M. Ussher, "Pathologizing Premenstrual Change," *Managing the Monstrous Feminine* (London: Routledge, 2006).

8. Insurance Institute for Highway Safety, "General Statistics: Gender," accessed August 22, 2016, http://www.iihs.org/iihs/topics/t/general-statistics/fatalityfacts/gender.

9. A. O'Connor, "Katharina Dalton, Expert on PMS, Dies at 87," *New York Times*, September 28, 2004, http://www.nytimes.com/2004/09/28/science/katharina-dalton-expert-on-pms-dies-at-87.html.

10. B. L. Jacobs, "PMS HAHAcronym: Perpetuating Male Superiority."

11. J. C. Chrisler and K. B. Levy, "The Media Construct a Menstrual Monster: A Content Analysis of PMS Articles in the Popular Press," *Women and Health* 16, no. 2 (1990): 89–104. doi:10.1300/j013v16n02_07.

12. M. Gurevich, "Rethinking the Label," *Women and Health* 23, no. 2 (1995): 67–98. doi:10.1300/j013v23n02_05.

13. Ibid.

14. A. L. Stanton, M. Lobel, S. Sears, and R. S. Deluca, "Psychosocial Aspects of Selected Issues in Women's Reproductive Health: Current Status and Future Directions." *Journal of Consulting and Clinical Psychology* 70, no. 3 (2002): 751–70. doi:10.1037/0022-006x.70.3.751.

15. D. T. Campbell, J. C. Stanley, and N. L. Gage, *Experimental and Quasi-Experimental Designs for Research* (Chicago: R. McNally, 1963).

16. J. C. Chrisler et al., "The Media Construct a Menstrual Monster."

17. J. C. Chrisler, I. K. Johnston, N. M. Champagne, and K. E. Preston, "Menstrual Joy: The Construct and Its Consequences," *Psychology of Women Quarterly* 18, no. 3 (1994): 375–87. doi:10.1111/j.1471–6402.1994.tb00461.x.

18. J. C. Chrisler, "PMS as a Culture-Bound Syndrome," *Lectures on the Psychology of Women*, ed. J. C. Chrisler, C. Golden, and P. D. Rozee (New York: McGraw-Hill. 2003): 165.

19. M. Yu, X. Zhu, J. Li, D. Oakley, and N. E. Reame, "Perimenstrual Symptoms Among Chinese Women in an Urban Area of China," *Health Care for Women International* 17, no. 2 (1996): 161–72. doi:10.1080/07399339609516230.

20. S. K. Chaturvedi, P. Chandra, G. Gururaj, C. Y. Sudarshan, M. B. Beena, and D. Panadian, "Prevalence of Premenstrual Symptoms and Syndromes: Preliminary Observations," *NIMHANS Journal* 12 (1994): 9–14.

21. K. D. Hoerster, J. C. Chrisler, and J. Gorman Rose. "Attitudes Toward and Experience with Menstruation in the US and India," *Women and Health* 38, no. 3 (2003): 77–95. doi:10.1300/j013v38n03_06.

22. A. O. Adewuya, O. M. Loto, and T. A. Adewumi, "Premenstrual Dysphoric Disorder Amongst Nigerian University Students: Prevalence, Comorbid Conditions, and Correlates," *Archives of Women's Mental Health* 11, no. 1 (2008): 13–18. doi:10.1007/s00737 –008–0213–4; L. S. Cohen, C. N. Soares, M. W. Otto, B. H. Sweeney, R. F. Liberman, and B. L. Harlow, "Prevalence and Predictors of Premenstrual Dysphoric Disorder (PMDD) in Older Premenopausal Women." *Journal of Affective Disorders* 70, no. 2 (2002): 125–32. doi:10.1016/s0165–0327(01)00458-x; S. Gehlert, I. H. Song, C. H. Chang, and S. A. Hartlage. "The Prevalence of Premenstrual Dysphoric Disorder." *Psychological Medicine* 39 (2009): 129–36; S. Tschudin, P. C. Bertea, and E. Zemp, "Prevalence and Predictors of Premenstrual Syndrome and Premenstrual Dysphoric Disorder in a Population-Based Sample." *Archives of Women's Mental Health* 13, no. 6 (2010): 485–94. doi:10.1007/s00737–010–0165–3.

23. J. M. McFarlane and T. M. Williams, "Placing Premenstrual Syndrome in Perspective," *Psychology of Women Quarterly* 18, no. 3 (1994): 339–73. doi:10.1111/j.1471–6402.1994. tb00460.x.

24. M. W. Matlin, "From Menarche to Menopause"; A. Offman, and P. J. Kleinplatz, "Does PMDD Belong in the DSM: Challenging the Medicalization of Women's Bodies," *The Canadian Journal of Human Sexuality* 13 (2004): 17–27.

25. A. E. Figert, *Women and the Ownership of PMS*.

26. J. Cunningham, K. A. Yonkers, S. O'Brien, and E. Eriksson, "Update on Research and Treatment of Premenstrual Dysphoric Disorder," *Harvard Review of Psychiatry* 17, no. 2 (2009): 120–37. doi:10.1080/10673220902891836.

27. A. E. Figert, *Women and the Ownership of PMS*.

28. C. A. Etaugh and J. S. Bridges, "Middle Adulthood: Physical Development and Health," *The Psychology of Women: A Lifespan Perspective* (Boston: Pearson, 2004): 342–43; C. Tavris, *The Mismeasure of Woman* (New York: Simon & Schuster, 1992).

29. B. Ehrenreich and D. English, "Witches, Healers, and Gentlemen Doctors," *For Her Own Good: Two Centuries of the Experts' Advice to Women* (New York: Anchor, 2005).

30. J. M. Metzl, "'Mother's Little Helper': The Crisis of Psychoanalysis and the Miltown Resolution." *Gender and History* 15, no. 2 (2003): 228–55. doi:10.1111/1468–0424.00300.

31. P. Chesler, *Women and Madness* (Garden City, NY: Doubleday, 1972): 284–99.

32. M. W. Matlin, "From Menarche to Menopause."

33. M. M. Kimball, "Feminists Rethink Gender," *About Psychology: Essays at the Crossroads of History, Theory, and Philosophy*, ed. D. B. Hill and M. J. Kral (Albany: State University of New York Press, 2003).

34. J. L. Sanders, "A Distinct Language and a Historic Pendulum: The Evolution of the Diagnostic and Statistical Manual of Mental Disorders," *Archives of Psychiatric Nursing* 25, no. 6 (2011): 394–403. doi:10.1016/j.apnu.2010.10.002.

35. A. E. Figert, *Women and the Ownership of PMS*.

36. C. Silverstein, "History of Treatment," *Textbook of Homosexuality and Mental Health*, ed. R. Cabaj (Arlington, VA: American Psychiatric Association, 1996): 3–16.

37. A. E. Figert, *Women and the Ownership of PMS*.

38. A. Offman and P. J. Kleinplatz, "Does PMDD Belong in the DSM: Challenging the Medicalization of Women's Bodies," *The Canadian Journal of Human Sexuality* 13 (2004): 17–27.

39. A. J. Frances, "DSM 5 Is Guide Not Bible—Ignore Its Ten Worst Changes." *Psychology Today*. December 2, 2012, https://www.psychologytoday.com/blog/dsm5-in-distress /201212/dsm-5-is-guide-not-bible-ignore-its-ten-worst-changes.

40. G. Greenberg, "The DSM's Troubled Revision," *New York Times*, January 29, 2012.

41. R. S. Rosenberg, "Abnormal Is the New Normal: Why Will Half of the U.S. Population Have a Diagnosable Mental Disorder?" *Slate*. April 12, 2013, http://www.slate.com /articles/health_and_science/medical_examiner/2013/04/diagnostic_and_statistical _manual_fifth_edition_why_will_half_the_u_s_population.html.

42. J. Wieczner, "Drug Companies Look to Profit from DSM 5," *Market Watch*, June 5, 2013, http://www.marketwatch.com/story/new-psych-manual-could-create-drug-wind falls-2013-06-05.

43. Ibid.

44. G. T. Schumock, E. C. Li, K. J. Suda, L. M. Matusiak, R. J. Hunkler, L. C. Vermeulen, and J. M. Hoffman, "National Trends in Prescription Drug Expenditures and Projections for 2014," *American Journal of Health-System Pharmacy* 71, no. 6 (2014): 482–99. doi:10.2146/ajhp130767.

45. N. Tadena, "The Most Medicated States," *Forbes*. August 16, 2010, http://www.forbes .com/2010/08/16/medications-pharmaceuticals-drugs-medicine-lifestyle-health-rx .html.

46. R. L. Kravitz, R. M. Epstein, M. D. Feldman, C. E. Franz, R. Azari, M. S. Wilkes, L. Hinton, and P. Franks, "Influence of Patients' Requests for Direct-To-Consumer Advertised Antidepressants: A Randomized Controlled Trial," *JAMA* 293, no. 16 (2005): 1995–2002.

47. D. C. Jain, and J. G. Conley, "Patent Expiry and Pharmaceutical Market Opportunities at the Nexus of Pricing and Innovation Policy," *Innovation and Marketing in the Pharmaceutical Industry: Emerging Practices, Research, and Policies*, ed. M. Ding, J. Eliashburg, and S. Stremersch (New York: Springer, 2014): 279.

48. J. Endicott, J. Amsterdam, E. Eriksson, et al., "Is Premenstrual Dysphoric Disorder a Distinct Clinical Entity?," *Journal of Women's Health and Gender-Based Medicine* 8, no. 5 (1999): 663–679.

49. P. J. Caplan, "The Debate About PMDD and Sarafem." *Women and Therapy* 27, no. 3–4 (2004): 55–67. doi:10.1300/j015v27n03_05.

50. J. C. Chrisler, and P. J. Caplan, "The Strange Case of Dr. Jekyll and Ms. Hyde: How PMS Became a Cultural Phenomenon and a Psychiatric Disorder," *Annual Review of Sex Research* 13 (2002): 274–306.

51. N. Tadena, "The Most Medicated States," *Forbes*.

52. J. C. Chrisler et al., "The Strange Case of Dr. Jekyll and Ms. Hyde"; R. Moynihan and Alan Cassels, *Selling Sickness: How the World's Biggest Pharmaceutical Companies Are Turning Us All into Patients* (New York: Nation Books, 2005).

53. J. Cunningham et al., "Update on Research and Treatment of Premenstrual Dysphoric Disorder."

54. J. Bancroft and Dilys Rennie, "The Impact of Oral Contraceptives on the Experience of Perimenstrual Mood, Clumsiness, Food Craving and Other Symptoms," *Journal of Psychosomatic Research* 37, no. 2 (1993): 195–202. doi:10.1016/0022–3999(93)90086-u; C. A. Graham and B. B. Sherwin. "A Prospective Treatment Study of Premenstrual Symptoms Using a Triphasic Oral Contraceptive," *Journal of Psychosomatic Research* 36, no. 3 (1992): 257–66. doi:10.1016/0022–3999(92)90090-o.

55. US Dept. of Health and Human Services, "Code of Federal Regulations, Title 21," April 1, 2016, http://www.accessdata.fda.gov/scripts/cdrh/cfdocs/cfCFR/CFRSearch .cfm?FR=860.7.

56. C. Tavris, *The Mismeasure of Woman.*

57. M. Bush, "Midol Makes a Game of Marketing to Teenage Girls," *DM News*, April 27, 2001, http://www.dmnews.com/midol-makes-a-game-of-marketing-to-teen-girls/article /72436/.

58. A. Alexander, "Niche Brands: Top 100," *Drugstore News*, May 13, 2013, http://www .drugstorenews.com/sites/drugstorenews.com/files/051313_NicheBrands_ONLINE .pdf.

59. See http://www.berkeleywellness.com/.

60. J. Cunningham et al., "Update on Research and Treatment of Premenstrual Dysphoric Disorder."

61. For a review see E. J. Frackiewicz and Thomas M. Shiovitz, "Evaluation and Management of Premenstrual Syndrome and Premenstrual Dysphoric Disorder," *Journal of the American Pharmaceutical Association* (1996) 41, no. 3 (2001): 437–47. doi:10.1016/ s1086–5802(16)31257–8.

62. M. L. Hardy, "Herbs of Special Interest to Women," *Journal of the American Pharmaceutical Association* (1996) 40, no. 2 (2000): 234–42. doi:10.1016/s1086–5802(16)31064–6.

63. See https://periodvitamin.com/.

64. J. C. Chrisler et al., "The Strange Case of Dr. Jekyll and Ms. Hyde"; M. Gurevich, "Rethinking the Label," *Women and Health* 23, no. 2 (1995): 67–98. doi:10.1300/j013 v23n02_05.

65. See, for example, http://www.vancouverwashingtonchiropractor.com/pms/

66. See http://naturopathicdoc.com/

67. See http://www.amenclinics.com/

68. J. Silver-Greenberg, "Patients Mired in Costly Credit from Doctors," *New York Times*, October 13, 2013, http://www.nytimes.com/2013/10/14/business/economy/patients-mired-in-costly-credit-from-doctors.html?pagewanted=all.

## Chapter 3: Keeping Women Down, Each and Every Month

1. As quoted in K. B. Golden, *Nietzsche and Disembodiment: Discerning Bodies and Non-Dualism* (Albany: State University of New York Press, 2006): 56.

2. B. L. Jacobs, "PMS HAHAcronym: Perpetuating Male Superiority."

3. Ibid.

4.  S. Laws, "The Sexual Politics of Pre-menstrual Tension," *Women's Studies International Forum* 6, no. 1 (1983): 19–31. doi:10.1016/0277-5395(83)90084-5.

5.  J. M. Ussher, and J. Perz, "Empathy, Egalitarianism and Emotion Work in the Relational Negotiation of PMS: The Experience of Women in Lesbian Relationships," *Feminism and Psychology* 18, no. 1 (2008): 87–111. doi:10.1177/0959353507084954.

6.  B. Ehrenreich, et al., "Witches, Healers, and Gentlemen Doctors."

7.  B. Welter, "The Cult of True Womanhood: 1820–1860," *Domestic Ideology and Domestic Work*, ed. N. F. Cott (New York: Aldine De Gruyter, 1992) doi:10.1515/978311 0968859.48.

8.  C. H. Gilman [Mrs. Clarissa Parkard, pseud.], *Recollections of a Housekeeeper* (New York: Harper & Brothers, 1834): 122.

9.  As quoted in B. Welter, "The Cult of True Womanhood," 162.

10. C. P. Gilman et al., *The Yellow Wallpaper.* (Boston: Bedford Books, 1998) originally published in 1913.

11. E. Martin, "Premenstrual Syndrome, Work, Discipline, and Anger," *The Woman in the Body: A Cultural Analysis of Reproduction* (Boston, MA: Beacon Press, 1987): 113–83.

12. C. Tavris, *The Mismeasure of Woman.*

13. G. H. Seward, "Psychological Effects of the Menstrual Cycle on Women Workers," *Psychological Bulletin* 41, no. 2 (1944): 90–102. doi:10.1037/h0057779.

14. E. Martin, "Premenstrual Syndrome, Work, Discipline, and Anger."

15. Ibid.

16. H. N. Fullerton, Jr., "Labor Force Participation: 75 Years of Change, 1950–98 and 1998–2025," *Monthly Labor Review* 122 (1999): 3.

17. E. Rome, "Premenstrual Syndrome (PMS) Examined through a Feminist Lens," *Culture, Society, and Menstruation,* ed. V. Olsen and N. F. Woods (Washington, DC: Hemisphere Publishing Corporation, 1986): 145–51.

18. E. Martin, "Premenstrual Syndrome, Work, Discipline, and Anger."

19. S. Laws, "The Sexual Politics of Pre-menstrual Tension."

20. S. Faludi, *Backlash: The Undeclared War against American Women* (New York: Crown, 1991).

21. Ehrenreich, B. et al., "Witches, Healers, and Gentlemen Doctors."

22. J. C. Chrisler et al., "The Strange Case of Dr. Jekyll and Ms. Hyde."

23. US Department of Labor, "Women in the Labor Force in 2010," January 2011, https://www.dol.gov/wb/factsheets/Qf-laborforce-10.htm.

24. M. W. Matlin, "Women and Work," *The Psychology of Women* (Boston: Cengage Learning, 2011): 243.

25. J. M. Ussher, et al., "Empathy, Egalitarianism, and Emotion Work in the Relational Negotiation of PMS."

26. M. Gurevich, "Rethinking the Label," *Women and Health* 23, no. 2 (1995): 67–98. doi:10.1300/j013v23n02_05.

27. Bureau of Labor Statistics, "American Time Use Survey," US Deptartment of Labor, accessed October 2, 2016, http://www.bls.gov/TUS/CHARTS/HOUSEHOLD.HTM.

28. J. M. Ussher et al., "Empathy, Egalitarianism, and Emotion Work in the Relational Negotiation of PMS."

29. J. C. Chrisler, "2007 Presidential Address: Fear of Losing Control: Power, Perfectionism, and the Psychology of Women," *Psychology of Women Quarterly* 32, no. 1 (2008): 1–12. doi:10.1111/j.1471–6402.2007.00402.x.

30. M. Gurevich, "Rethinking the Label."

31. L. Z. Tiedens, "Anger and Advancement Versus Sadness and Subjugation: The Effect of Negative Emotion Expressions on Social Status Conferral," *Journal of Personality and Social Psychology* 80, no. 1 (2001): 86–94. doi:10.1037//0022–3514.80.1.86.

32. V. L. Brescoll and Eric Luis Uhlmann, "Can an Angry Woman Get Ahead? Status Conferral, Gender, and Expression of Emotion in the Workplace," *Psychological Science* 19, no. 3 (2008): 268–75. doi:10.1111/j.1467–9280.2008.02079.x.

33. For a review see N. Praill, A. A. González-Prendes, and P. Kernsmith, "An Exploration of the Relationships Between Attitudes Towards Anger Expression and Personal Style of Anger Expression in Women in the USA and Canada," *Issues in Mental Health Nursing* 36, no. 6 (2015): 397–406.

34. C. Z. Stearns and P. N. Stearns, *Anger: The Struggle for Emotional Control in America's History* (Chicago: University of Chicago Press, 1989).

35. D. L. Cox and S. St. Clair, "A New Perspective on Women's Anger: Therapy Through the Lens of Anger Diversion," *Women and Therapy* 28, no. 2 (2005): 77–90.

36. J. M. Ussher et al., "Empathy, Egalitarianism, and Emotion Work in the Relational Negotiation of PMS."

37. Ibid.

38. J. J. Bigner, "Gay and Lesbian Families," *Handbook of Family Development and Intervention*, ed. W. C. Nichols, M.S. Pace-Nichols, D. S. Becvar, and A. Y. Napier (New York: John Wiley and Sons, 2000): 279–98.; N. Toder, "Lesbian Couples in Particular," *Positively Gay: New Approaches to Gay and Lesbian Life*, ed. B. Berzon (Berkeley, CA: Celestial Arts, 1992): 50–63; N. S. Eldridge and L. A. Gilbert, "Correlates Of Relationship Satisfaction In Lesbian Couples," *Psychology of Women Quarterly* 14, no. 1 (1990): 43–62. doi:10.1111/j.1471–6402.1990.tb00004.x.

# Chapter 4: The "Significantly" Impaired Preggo

1. T. Sagher, "The Slutty Pumpkin Returns," *How I Met Your Mother*, CBS, aired October 31, 2011.

2. B. Karlin, "When a Tree Falls," *Modern Family*, ABC, aired November 28, 2012.

3. H. E. Murkoff and S. Mazel, *What to Expect When You're Expecting* (New York: Workman Publications, 2008): 214.

4. H. P. Kennedy, K. Nardini, R. Mcleod-Waldo, and L. Ennis, "Top-Selling Childbirth Advice Books: A Discourse Analysis," *Birth* 36, no. 4 (2009): 318–24. doi:10.1111/j.1523 –536x.2009.00359.x.

5. R. Crawley, S. Grant, and K. Hinshaw, "Cognitive Changes in Pregnancy: Mild Decline or Societal Stereotype?" *Applied Cognitive Psychology* 22, no. 8 (2008): 1142–162. doi:10.1002/acp.1427.

6.   J. Buckwalter, D. K. Buckwalter, B. W. Bluestein, and F. Z. Stanczyk, "Chapter 22 Pregnancy and Postpartum: Changes in Cognition and Mood," *Progress in Brain Research The Maternal Brain* (2001): 303–19. doi:10.1016/s0079–6123(01)33023–6; R. A. Crawley, K. Dennison, and C. Carter, "Cognition in Pregnancy and the First Year Post-partum," *Psychology and Psychotherapy: Theory, Research and Practice* 76, no. 1 (2003): 69–84. doi:10.1348/14760830260569265; R. H. deGroot, E. F. P. M. Vuurman, G. Hornstra, and J. Jolles, "Differences in Cognitive Performance during Pregnancy and Early Motherhood," *Psychological Medicine* 36, no. 07 (2006): 1023. doi:10.1017/s 0033291706007380.

7.   R. H. deGroot, J. J. Adam, and G. Hornstra, "Selective Attention Deficits during Human Pregnancy," *Neuroscience Letters* 340, no. 1 (2003): 21–24. doi:10.1016/s0304–3940(03)00034-x.

8.   J. Buckwalter et al., "Chapter 22 Pregnancy and Postpartum."

9.   J. F. Henry and Barbara B. Sherwin, "Hormones and Cognitive Functioning during Late Pregnancy and Postpartum: A Longitudinal Study," *Behavioral Neuroscience* 126, no. 1 (2012): 73–85. doi:10.1037/a0025540.

10.   H. E. Murkoff et al., *What to Expect When You're Expecting.*

11.   V. Iovine, *The Girlfriends' Guide to Pregnancy: Or Everything Your Doctor Won't Tell You* (New York: Pocket Books, 1995).

12.   A. C. Guyton and J. E. Hall, "Pregnancy and Lactation," *Textbook of Medical Physiology,* (Philadelphia: W.B. Saunders Company, 2000): 948–49.

13.   "Conception, Pregnancy, and Fetal Development," *Medical Physiology,* ed. G. A. Tanner and R. A. Rhoades (Baltimore: Lippincott, Williams, & Wilkins, 1995): 784–86.

14.   J.R. W. Fisher, M. Cabral De Mello, and T. Isutzu, "Pregnancy, Childbirth, and the Postpartum Year," *Mental Health Aspects of Women's Reproductive Health: A Global Review of the Literature* (Geneva: World Health Organization and the United Nations Population Fund, 2009).

15.   M. W. Matlin, "Pregnancy, Childbirth, and Motherhood," *The Psychology of Women;* A. L. Stanton et al., "Psychosocial Aspects of Selected Issues in Women's Reproductive Health."

16.   Ibid.

17.   H. Skouteris, R. Carr, E. H. Wertheim, S. J. Paxton, and D. Duncombe, "A Prospective Study of Factors That Lead to Body Dissatisfaction During Pregnancy," *Body Image* 2, no. 4 (2005): 347–61. doi:10.1016/j.bodyim.2005.09.002.

18.   D. M. Mitnick, R. E. Heyman, and A. M. Smith Slep, "Changes in Relationship Satisfaction across the Transition to Parenthood: A Meta-analysis," *Journal of Family Psychology* 23, no. 6 (2009): 848–52. doi:10.1037/a0017004.

19.   S. Knapton, "'Baby Brain' Really Does Exist, Say Scientists," *Telegraph,* May 7, 2014, http://www.telegraph.co.uk/news/science/science-news/10812090/Baby-brain-really -does-exist-say-scientists.html.

20.   N. E. Hurt, "Legitimizing 'Baby Brain': Tracing a Rhetoric of Significance Through Science and the Mass Media," *Communication and Critical/Cultural Studies* 8, no. 4 (2011): 376–98. doi:10.1080/14791420.2011.619202.

21.   J. D. Henry and P. G. Rendell, "A Review of the Impact of Pregnancy on Memory Function," *Journal of Clinical and Experimental Neuropsychology* 29, no. 8 (2007): 793–803. doi:10.1080/13803390701612209.

22. J. W. Cohen, *Statistical Power Analysis for the Behavioral Sciences* (New York: Academic Press, 1977).

23. N. E. Hurt, "Legitimizing 'Baby Brain.'"

24. J.R. W. Fisher et al., "Pregnancy, Childbirth, and the Postpartum Year."

# Chapter 5: A Pregnant Body Rules a Woman

1. E. Becker, *Escape from Evil* (New York: Free Press, 1975).

2. S. De Beauvoir, *The Second Sex* (New York: Alfred Knopf, 1952) xxi-xxii.

3. Ehrenreich, B. et al., "Witches, Healers, and Gentlemen Doctors."

4. K.K. Barker, "A Ship upon a Stormy Sea: The Medicalization of Pregnancy," *Social Science and Medicine* 47, no. 8 (1998): 1067–076. doi:10.1016/s0277–9536(98)00155-5.

5. J. Waller, "Lessons from the History of Medicine," *Journal of Investigative Surgery* 21, no. 2 (2008): 53–56. doi:10.1080/08941930801986459.

6. R. Davis-Floyd, *Birth as an American Rite of Passage* (Berkeley: University of California Press, 2004).

7. K. M. Dewbury, D. Cosgrove, and P. Farrant, *Ultrasound in Obstetrics and Gynecology, Vol. 3* (London: Churchill Livingstone, 2004).

8. J. S. Abramowicz, "Benefits and Risks of Ultrasound in Pregnancy," *Seminars in Perinatology* 37, no. 5 (2013): 295–300. doi:10.1053/j.semperi.2013.06.004.

9. American College of Obstetricians and Gynecologists, "Guidelines for Diagnostic Imaging during Pregnancy and Lactation," February 2016, http://www.acog.org/Resources-And-Publications/Committee-Opinions/Committee-on-Obstetric-Practice/Guidelines-for-Diagnostic-Imaging-During-Pregnancy-and-Lactation.

10. D. F. O'Keeffe and Alfred Abuhamad, "Obstetric Ultrasound Utilization in the United States: Data from Various Health Plans," *Seminars in Perinatology* 37, no. 5 (2013): 292–94. doi:10.1053/j.semperi.2013.06.003.

11. J. P. Newnham, S. F. Evans, C. A. Michael, F. J. Stanley, and L. I. Landau, "Effects of Frequent Ultrasound during Pregnancy: A Randomized Controlled Trial," *The Lancet* 342, no. 8876 (1993): 887–91. doi:10.1016/0140–6736(93)91944-h.

12. J. S. Abramowicz, "Benefits and Risks of Ultrasound in Pregnancy."

13. US Food and Drug Administration, "Fetal Keepsake Videos," May 12, 2015, http://www.fda.gov/MedicalDevices/Safety/AlertsandNotices/PatientAlerts/ucm064756.htm.

14. E. Asher, S. Dvir, D. S. Seidman, S. Greenberg-Dotan, A. Kedem, B. Sheizaf, and H. Reuveni, "Defensive Medicine among Obstetricians and Gynecologists in Tertiary Hospitals," *PLOS ONE* 8, no. 3 (2013). doi:10.1371/journal.pone.0057108.

15. H. K. Hallgrimsdottir and B. E. Benner, "'Knowledge Is Power': Risk and the Moral Responsibilities of the Expectant Mother at the Turn of the Twentieth Century," *Health, Risk and Society* 16, no. 1 (2013): 7–21. doi:10.1080/13698575.2013.866216.

16. S. A. Shaw, "Chicken of the Sea," *New York Times*, July 15, 2015, http://www.nytimes.com/2007/07/15/opinion/15shaw.html?_r=0.

17. A. D. Lyerly, L. M. Mitchell, E. M. Armstrong, L. H. Harris, R. Kukla, M. Kuppermann, and M. O. Little, "Risk and the Pregnant Body," *Hastings Center Report* 39, no. 6 (2009): 34–42. doi:10.1353/hcr.0.0211.

18. National Vital Statistics Reports, "Births: Final Data for 2013," January 15, 2015, http://www.cdc.gov/nchs/data/nvsr/nvsr64/nvsr64_01.pdf.

19. A. L. Chan, M. M. Juarez, N. Gidwani, and T. E. Albertson, "Management of Critical Asthma Syndrome During Pregnancy," *Clinical Reviews in Allergy and Immunology* 48, no. 1 (2013): 45–53. doi:10.1007/s12016–013–8397–4; A. D. Lyerly et al. "Risk and the Pregnant Body."

20. K. L. Lawson, "Perceptions of Deservedness of Social Aid as a Function of Prenatal Diagnostic Testing." *Journal of Applied Social Psychology* 33, no. 1 (2003): 76–90. doi:10.1111/j.1559–1816.2003.tb02074.x.

21. S.M. Woods, J.L. Melville, Y. Guo, M.Y. Fan, and A. Gavin, "Psychosocial Stress during Pregnancy," *Obstetric Anesthesia Digest* 30, no. 4 (2010): 237. doi:10.1097/01.aoa.0000389617.09252.47.

22. E.J. H. Mulder, P. G. Robles De Medina, A. C. Huizink, B. R. H. Van Den Bergh, J. K. Buitelaar, and G. H. A. Visser, "Prenatal Maternal Stress: Effects on Pregnancy and the (Unborn) Child," *Early Human Development* 70, no. 1–2 (2002): 3–14. doi:10.1016/s0378–3782(02)00075–0.

23. T. Wainstock, L. Lerner-Geva, S. Glasser, I. Shoham-Vardi, and E. Y. Anteby, "Prenatal Stress and Risk of Spontaneous Abortion," *Psychosomatic Medicine* 75, no. 3 (2013): 228–35. doi:10.1097/psy.0b013e318280f5f3.

24. C. D. Schetter, "Psychological Science on Pregnancy: Stress Processes, Biopsychosocial Models, and Emerging Research Issues." *Annual Review of Psychology* 62, no. 1 (2011): 531-58. doi:10.1146/annurev.psych.031809.130727; M. Tegethoff, N. Greene, J. Olsen, E. Schaffner, and G. Meinlschmidt, "Stress During Pregnancy and Offspring Pediatric Disease: A National Cohort Study." *Environmental Health Perspectives* 119, no. 11 (2011): 1647-652. doi:10.1289/ehp.1003253.

25. For a review see P. L. Marca-Ghaemmaghami and U. Ehlert, "Stress During Pregnancy," *European Psychologist* 20, no. 2 (2015): 102–19. doi:10.1027/1016–9040/a000195.

26. M. M. Butler, L. Sheehy, M. Kington, M. C. Walsh, M. C. Brosnan, M. Murphy, C. Naughton, J. Drennan, and T. Barry, "Evaluating Midwife-led Antenatal Care: Choice, Experience, Effectiveness, and Preparation for Pregnancy," *Midwifery* 31, no. 4 (2015): 418–25. doi:10.1016/j.midw.2014.12.002.

27. J. Sandall, H. Soltani, S. Gates, A. Shennan, and D. Devane, "Midwife-Led Continuity Models Versus Other Models of Care for Childbearing Women," *Cochrane Database of Systematic Reviews 2013*, no. 8. doi:10.1002/14651858.CD004667.pub3

28. J. A. Martin, B. E. Hamilton, M. J. Osterman, S. C. Curtin, and T. J. Matthews, "Births: Final Data for 2013." *National Vital Statistics Reports: from the Centers for Disease Control and Prevention, National Center for Health Statistics, National Vital Statistics System* 64, no. 1 (2015): 1-65.

29. L. L. Laughlin, "Maternity Leave and Employment Patterns of First-Time Mothers: 1961–2008." US Department of Commerce, Economics, and Statistics Administration (US Census Bureau, 2011); Fried, M. *Taking Time: Parental Leave Policy and Corporate Culture* (Philadelphia: Temple University Press, 1998).

30. A. M. Koenig, A. H. Eagly, and A. A. Mitchell. "Are Leader Stereotypes Masculine? A Meta-Analysis of Three Research Paradigms," *Psychological Bulletin* (2011). doi:10.1037/e617292010–001.

31. A. B. Fox, and D. M. Quinn, "Pregnant Women at Work: The Role of Stigma in Predicting Women's Intended Exit from the Workforce," *Psychology of Women Quarterly* 39, no. 2 (2014): 226–42. doi:10.1177/0361684314552653; E. B. King and W. E. Botsford, "Managing Pregnancy Disclosures: Understanding and Overcoming the Challenges of Expectant Motherhood at Work," *Human Resource Management Review* 19, no. 4 (2009): 314–23. doi:10.1016/j.hrmr.2009.03.003.

32. C. L. Ridgeway and S. J. Correll, "Motherhood as a Status Characteristic," *Journal of Social Issues* 60, no. 4 (2004): 683–700. doi:10.1111/j.0022–4537.2004.00380.x.

33. J. Williams, *Unbending Gender: Why Family and Work Conflict and What to Do about It* (Oxford: Oxford University Press, 2000).

34. A. H. Eagly, and S. J. Karau, "Role Congruity Theory of Prejudice toward Female Leaders," *Psychological Review* 109, no. 3 (2002): 573–98. doi:10.1037//0033–295x .109.3.573.

35. M. Heilman, "Sex Bias in Work Settings: The Lack of Fit Model," *Research in Organizational Behavior* 5 (1983): 269–98.

36. M. R. Hebl, E. B. King, P. Glick, S. L. Singletary, and S. Kazama, "Hostile and Benevolent Reactions toward Pregnant Women: Complementary Interpersonal Punishments and Rewards That Maintain Traditional Roles," *Journal of Applied Psychology* 92, no. 6 (2007): 1499–511. doi:10.1037/0021–9010.92.6.1499.

37. A. B. Fox and D. M. Quinn, "Pregnant Women at Work: The Role of Stigma in Predicting Women's Intended Exit from the Workforce," *Psychology of Women Quarterly* 39, no. 2 (2014): 226–42. doi:10.1177/0361684314552653.

38. T. D. Johnson, "Maternity Leave and Employment Patterns: 2001–2003," *Current Population Report* (Washington, DC: US Census Bureau, 2007): 70–113.

39. J. A Halpert and J. Hickman Burg, "Mixed Messages: Coworker Responses to the Pregnant Employee," *Journal of Business and Psychology* 12, no. 2 (1997): 241–253.

40. M. R. Hebl, E. B. King, P. Glick, S. L. Singletary, and S. Kazama, "Hostile and Benevolent Reactions toward Pregnant Women: Complementary Interpersonal Punishments and Rewards That Maintain Traditional Roles," *Journal of Applied Psychology* 92, no. 6 (2007): 1499–511. doi:10.1037/0021–9010.92.6.1499.

41. J. D. Bragger, E. Kutcher, J. Morgan, and P. Firth, "The Effects of the Structured Interview on Reducing Biases against Pregnant Job Applicants," *Sex Roles* 46 (2002): 215–26.

42. J. Cunningham and T. H. Macan, "Effects of Applicant Pregnancy on Hiring Decisions and Interview Ratings," *Sex Roles* 57, no. 7 (2007): 497–508. doi:10.1007/s11199–007 –9279–0.

43. A. Scaccia, "The Face of Pregnancy Discrimination," *Rewire*, May 1, 2013, https:// rewire.news/article/2013/05/01/the-face-of-pregnancy-discrimination/.

44. Equal Employment Opportunity Commission, "University of Milwaukee to Pay $37,500 in EEOC Pregnancy Discrimination Suit," March 14, 2013, https://www.eeoc.gov //eeoc/newsroom/release/3–14–13a.cfm.

45. Equal Employment Opportunity Commission, "Fact Sheet on Recent EEOC Pregnancy Discrimination Litigation," accessed September 4, 2016, https://www.eeoc.gov /laws/guidance/pregnancy_fact_sheet_litigation.cfm.

46. L. M. Little, V. S. Major, A. S. Hinojosa, and D. L. Nelson, "Professional Image Maintenance: How Women Navigate Pregnancy in the Workplace," *Academy of Management Journal* 58, no. 1 (2015): 8–37.

47. T. J. Mathews and B. E. Hamilton, "First Births to Older Women Continue to Rise," *National Center for Health Statistics Data Brief* 152 (2014): 1–8.

48. A. R. Miller, "The Effects of Motherhood Timing on Career Path," *Journal of Population Economics* 24, no. 3 (2009): 1071–100. doi:10.1007/s00148–009–0296-x.

49. M. Simonsen and Lars Skipper, "The Costs of Motherhood: An Analysis Using Matching Estimators," *Journal of Applied Econometrics* 21, no. 7 (2006): 919–34. doi:10.1002/jae.893; M. J. Budig and P. England, "The Wage Penalty for Motherhood," *American Sociological Review* 66, no. 2 (2001): 204. doi:10.2307/2657415.

50. For a review of all medical risks related to delayed childbearing see K. Benzies, S.Tough, K. Tofflemire, C. Frick, A. Faber, and C. Newburn-Cook, "Factors Influencing Women's Decisions About Timing of Motherhood," *Journal of Obstetric, Gynecologic and Neonatal Nursing* 35, no. 5 (2006): 625–33. doi:10.1111/j.1552–6909.2006.00079.x.

## Chapter 6: The Media's Perfect Postpartum Storm

1. For a review see M. W. O'Hara and K. L. Wisner, "Perinatal Mental Illness: Definition, Description and Aetiology," *Best Practice and Research Clinical Obstetrics & Gynaecology* 28, no. 1 (2014): 3–12.

2. "Those Mysterious Childbirth Blues," *Good Housekeeping*, May 1960: 165–66.

3. "Postpartum Depression," *WebMd.com*, accessed July 2, 2016.

4. J. Baxter, S. Buchler, F. Perales, and M. Western, "A Life-Changing Event: First Births and Men's and Women's Attitudes to Mothering and Gender Divisions of Labor," *Social Forces* 93, no. 3 (2015): 989–1014.

5. "Postpartum Depression," *MayoClinic.org*, accessed October 02, 2016.

6. L. Tigar, "11 Celebrity Moms Who Overcame Postpartum Depression," *Parents*, accessed October 02, 2016.

7. J. Fisher, M. Cabral de Mello, and T. Izutsu, "Mental Health Aspects of Pregnancy, Childbirth and the Postpartum Period," *Contemporary Topics in Women's Mental Health: Global Perspectives in a Changing Society* (Oxford: Wiley-Blackwell, 2009): 197–225; I. S. Yim, L. R. T. Stapleton, C. M. Guardino, J. Hahn-Holbrook, and C. D. Schetter, "Biological and Psychosocial Predictors of Postpartum Depression: Systematic Review and Call for Integration," *Clinical Psychology* 11, no. 1 (2015). 99.

8. L. Held and A. Rutherford, "Can't a Mother Sing the Blues? Postpartum Depression and the Construction of Motherhood in Late 20th-Century America," *History of Psychology* 15, no. 2 (2012): 107.

9. N. I. Gavin, B. N. Gaynes, K. N. Lohr, S. Meltzer-Brody, G. Gartlehner, and T. Swinson, "Perinatal Depression," *Obstetrics and Gynecology* 106, no. 5, Part 1 (2005): 1071–083. doi:10.1097/01.aog.0000183597.31630.db.

10. K. Eban, "Depression: Back to Life," *Working Mother*, November 14, 2008, http://www.workingmother.com/2008/11/work/depression-back-life

11. P. Belluck, "Panel Calls for Depression Screenings During and After Pregnancy," *New York Times,* January 26, 2016, http://www.nytimes.com/2016/01/27/health/post-partum-depression-test-epds-screening-guidelines.html?_r=0

12. "Postpartum Depression," *MayoClinic.org*, accessed October 02, 2016.

13. C. Teproff and B. Dupuy, "Police: Mother Blames Postpartum Depression for Trying to Kill Her Baby," *Miami Herald*, July 2, 2014.

14. K. Wallace, "Moms Who Need Mental Health Care the Most Aren't Getting It," *CNN.com*, November 2, 2015, http://www.cnn.com/2015/11/02/health/mothers-mental -health-postpartum-depression/.

15. A. Toufexis, "Behavior: Why Mothers Kill Their Babies, *Time*, June 20, 1988, http:// content.time.com/time/magazine/article/0,9171,967743,00.html.

16. C. L. Schanie, M. D. Pinto-Foltz, and M. C. Logsdon, "Analysis of Popular Press Articles Concerning Postpartum Depression: 1998–2006," *Issues in Mental Health Nursing* 29, no. 11 (2008): 1200–1216.

17. D. W. Denno, "Who Is Andrea Yates? A Short Story About Insanity," *Duke Journal of Gender Law and Policy* 10 (2003): 1–139.

18. Ibid.

19. M. Gamiz, "2 Tragic Cases Show Marked Contrasts," *Los Angeles Times: Monday Home Edition*, April 15, 2002, http://articles.latimes.com/2002/apr/15/local/me-adair15.

20. A. Quindlen, "Playing God On No Sleep," *Newsweek*, July 1, 2001, http://www.news week.com/playing-god-no-sleep-154643.

21. R. Hyman, "Medea of Suburbia: Andrea Yates, Maternal Infanticide, and the Insanity Defense," *Women's Studies Quarterly* 32, no. 3/4 (2004): 192–210.

22. "Baby Killer Andrea Yates Gets Off on Insanity Defense," *IndependentConservative. com*, July 26, 2006, http://www.independentconservative.com/2006/07/26/andrea _yates_beats_charges/.

23. S. May, "What Have We Done to Motherhood?" *Rightgrrl.com*, July 10, 2001, http:// www.rightgrrl.com/2001/yates.shtml.

24. A. Cohen, "How Andrea Yates Lives, and Lives with Herself, a Decade Later," *The Atlantic*, March 12, 2012, http://www.theatlantic.com/national/archive/2012/03 /how-andrea-yates-lives-and-lives-with-herself-a-decade-later/254302/.

## Chapter 7: That's Not Me Crying, It Must Be the Baby

1. B. Ehrenreich and D. English, "Motherhood as Pathology," *For Her Own Good: Two Centuries of the Experts' Advice to Women* (New York: Anchor, 2005).

2. C. Knudson-Martin and R. Silverstein, "Suffering in Silence: A Qualitative Meta-Data-Analysis of Postpartum Depression," *Journal of Marital and Family Therapy* 35, no. 2 (2009): 145–58. doi:10.1111/j.1752–0606.2009.00112.x.

3. M. W. O'Hara et al., "Perinatal Mental Illness: Definition, Description and Aetiology."

4. J.R. W. Fisher et al., "Pregnancy, Childbirth, and the Postpartum Year"; I. S. Yim et al., "Biological and Psychosocial Predictors of Postpartum Depression: Systematic Review and Call for Integration"; M. W. O'Hara and L. S. Segre, "Psychological Disorders of Pregnancy and the Postpartum," *Danforth's Obstetrics and Gynecology* (Philadelphia: Lippincott, Williams, and Wilkins, 2008).

5. M. W. O'Hara et al., "Psychological Disorders of Pregnancy and the Postpartum."

6. M. W. O'Hara et al., "Perinatal Mental Illness: Definition, Description and Aetiology."

7.  C. Chatzicharalampous, D. Rizos, P. Pliatsika, A. Leonardou, D. Hasiakos, I. Zervas, A. Alexandrou, M. Creatsa, S. Konidaris, and I. Lambrinoudaki, "Reproductive Hormones and Postpartum Mood Disturbances in Greek Women," *Gynecological Endocrinology* 27, no. 8 (2010): 543–50. doi:10.3109/09513590.2010.501886.

8.  M. Bloch, N. Rotenberg, D. Koren, and E. Klein, "Risk Factors for Early Postpartum Depressive Symptoms," *General Hospital Psychiatry* 28, no. 1 (2006): 3–8. doi:10.1016/j .genhosppsych.2005.08.006.

9.  J.R. W. Fisher et al., "Pregnancy, Childbirth, and the Postpartum Year."

10.  B. D. Howard, "The Emptiness of Postpartum Depression," *Goop.com*, accessed January 2, 2016, http://goop.com/bryce-dallas-howard-on-the-emptiness-of-postpartum -depression/.

11.  N. I. Gavin, B. N. Gaynes, K. N. Lohr, S. Meltzer-Brody, G. Gartlehner, and T. Swinson. "Perinatal Depression." Obstetrics & Gynecology 106, no. 5, Part 1 (2005): 1071– 083. doi:10.1097/01.aog.0000183597.31630.db.

12.  J.R. W. Fisher et al., "Pregnancy, Childbirth, and the Postpartum Year"; I. S. Yim et al., "Biological and Psychosocial Predictors of Postpartum Depression: Systematic Review and Call for Integration"; M. W. O'Hara, "Postpartum Depression: What We Know," *Journal of Clinical Psychology* 65, no. 12 (2009): 1258–269. doi:10.1002/jclp.20644.

13.  R. S. Deluca and M. Lobel, "Diminished Control and Unmet Expectations: Testing a Model of Adjustment to Unplanned Cesarean Delivery," *Analyses of Social Issues and Public Policy* 14, no. 1 (2014): 183–204. doi:10.1111/asap.12040.

14.  M. W. O'Hara, "Postpartum Depression: What We Know."

15.  J.R. W. Fisher et al., "Pregnancy, Childbirth, and the Postpartum Year."

16.  I. S. Yim et al., "Biological and Psychosocial Predictors of Postpartum Depression: Systematic Review and Call for Integration."

17  C. Monzon, T. L. Di Scala, and T. Pearlstein, "Postpartum Psychosis: Updates and Clinical Issues," *Psychiatric Times*, January 15, 2014, http://www.psychiatrictimes.com /special-reports/postpartum-psychosis-updates-and-clinical-issues.

18.  Ibid.

19.  A. Di Florio, S. Smith, and I. Jones, "Postpartum Psychosis," *The Obstetrician & Gynecologist* 15, no. 3 (2013): 145–150; J.R. W. Fisher et al., "Pregnancy, Childbirth, and the Postpartum Year."

20.  A. Young and J. Eberhard, "Evaluating Depressive Symptoms in Mania: A Naturalistic Study of Patients with Bipolar Disorder," *Neuropsychiatric Disease and Treatment*, 2015, 1137. doi:10.2147/ndt.s82532.

21.  A. Di Florio et al., "Postpartum Psychosis."

22.  K. A. Kendall-Tackett, *Depression in New Mothers: Causes, Consequences, and Treatment Alternatives* (New York: Haworth Maltreatment and Trauma Press, 2005).

23.  V. Lindahl, J. L. Pearson, and L. Colpe, "Prevalence of Suicidality during Pregnancy and the Postpartum," *Archives of Women's Mental Health* 8, no. 2 (2005): 77–87. doi:10.1007/s00737–005–0080–1.

24.  I. Engqvist and Kerstin Nilsson, "Experiences of the First Days of Postpartum Psychosis: An Interview Study with Women and Next of Kin in Sweden," *Issues in Mental Health Nursing* 34, no. 2 (2013): 82–89. doi:10.3109/01612840.2012.723301.

25. T. Field, D. E. Sandberg, R. Garcia, L. Guy, "Pregnancy Problems, Postpartum Depression, and Early Mother-Infant Interactions," *Developmental Psychology* 21, no. 6 (1985): 1152–156. doi:10.1037//0012–1649.21.6.1152.

26. M. W. O'Hara, "Postpartum Depression: What We Know."

27. K. A. Kendall-Tackett, *Depression in New Mothers.*

28. I. Luoma, T. Tamminen, P. Kaukonen, P. Laippala, K. Puura, R. Salmelin, and F. Almqvist, "Longitudinal Study of Maternal Depressive Symptoms and Child Well-Being," *Journal of the American Academy of Child and Adolescent Psychiatry* 40, no. 12 (2001): 1367–374. doi:10.1097/00004583–200112000–00006.

29. D. R. Forman, M. W. O'Hara, S. Stuart, L. L. Gorman, K. E. Larsen, and K. C. Coy, "Effective Treatment for Postpartum Depression Is Not Sufficient to Improve the Developing Mother–Child Relationship," *Development and Psychopathology* 19, no. 02 (2007). doi:10.1017/s0954579407070289.

30. K. A. Kendall-Tackett, *Depression in New Mothers.*

31. D. R. Forman et al., "Effective Treatment for Postpartum Depression Is Not Sufficient to Improve the Developing Mother–child Relationship."

32. I. Engqvist et al., "Experiences of the First Days of Postpartum Psychosis."

33. C. Monzon et al., "Postpartum Psychosis."

34. J. H. Harvey and A. Wenzel, *Close Romantic Relationships: Maintenance and Enhancement* (Mahwah, NJ: Lawrence Erlbaum Associates, 2001) 300–306.

35. J. Breslau, E. Miller, R. Jin, N. A. Sampson, J. Alonso, L. H. Andrade, E. J. Bromet, G. De Girolamo, K. Demyttenaere, J. Fayyad, A. Fukao, M. Galaon, O. Gureje, Y. He, H. R. Hinkov, C. Hu, V. Kovess-Masfety, H. Matschinger, M. E. Medina-Mora, J. Ormel, J. Posada-Villa, R. Sagar, K. M. Scott, and R. C. Kessler, "A Multinational Study of Mental Disorders, Marriage, and Divorce," *Acta Psychiatrica Scandinavica* 124, no. 6 (2011): 474–86. doi:10.1111/j.1600–0447.2011.01712.x.

36. S. B. McCabe and I. H. Gotlib, "Interactions of Couples With and Without a Depressed Spouse: Self-Report and Observations of Problem-Solving Situations," *Journal of Social and Personal Relationships* 10, no. 4 (1993): 589–99. doi:10.1177/0265407593104007.

37. H. A. O'Mahen, S. R.H Beach, and S. F. Banawan, "Depression in Marriage," *Close Romantic Relationships: Maintenance and Enhancement* ed. J. H. Harvey and A. Wenzel (Mahwah, NJ: Lawrence Erlbaum Associates, 2001): 299–320.

38. M. W. O'Hara, "Postpartum Depression: What We Know."

## Chapter 8: The Reputation of Menopause Precedes It

1. As quoted in L. Rosewarne, *Periods in Pop Culture.*

2. S. Sontag, "The Double Standard of Aging," *The Other Within Us: Feminist Explorations of Women and Aging,* ed. Marilyn Pearsall (Boulder, CO: Westview Press, 1997).

3. J. M. Ussher, "Menopause and the Ageing Body," *Managing the Monstrous Feminine,* (New York: Routledge, 2006): 145.

4. Last Fuckable Day. By Amy Schumer. Comedy Central, 2015. Television. http://www.cc.com/video-clips/a30bcg/inside-amy-schumer-last-f--kable-day---uncensored.

5. *TNIV Holy Bible* (Grand Rapids, MI: Zondervan, 2005).

6. R. Formanek, "Continuity and Change and 'the Change of Life': Premodern Views of the Menopause," *The Meanings of Menopause: Historical, Medical, and Cultural Perspectives* (London: Routledge, 1990): 3–42.

7. J. Oeppen and J. W. Vaupel, "Broken Limits to Life Expectancy," *Science* 296, no. 5570 (2002): 1029–1031.

8. B. Ehrenreich et al., *For her own good: Two centuries of the Experts' Advice to Women.*

9. J. A. Houck, *Hot and Bothered: Women, Medicine, and Menopause in Modern America.* (Cambridge, MA: Harvard University Press, 2006).

10. M. Lincoln, *You'll Live Through It: Facts About Menopause* (New York: Harper, 1950): 148.

11. J. A. Houck, *Hot and Bothered: Women, Medicine, and Menopause in Modern America,* 125.

12. R. A. Wilson and T. A. Wilson, "The Fate of the Nontreated Postmenopausal Woman: A Plea for the Maintenance of Adequate Estrogen from Puberty to the Grave," *Journal of the American Geriatrics Society* 11, no. 4 (1963): 347–362; R. A. Wilson, *Feminine Forever* (New York: M. Evans and Company, 1966).

13. E. S. Watkins, *The Estrogen Elixir: A History of Hormone Replacement Therapy in America* (Baltimore: Johns Hopkins University Press, 2007).

14. B. Seaman, *The Greatest Experiment Ever Performed on Women: Exploding the Estrogen Myth* (New York: Seven Stories Press, 2003): 49.

15 S. Munch, "The Women's Health Movement: Making Policy, 1970–1995," *Social Work in Health Care* 43, no. 1 (2006): 17–32.

16. A. C. Mastroianni, R. Faden, and D. Federman, *Women and Health Research: Ethical and Legal Issues of Including Women in Clinical Studies, Volume 1* (Washington, DC: The National Academies Press, 1994).

17. N. Singer and D. Wilson, "Menopause, as Brought to You by Big Pharma," *New York Times,* December 12, 2009, http://www.nytimes.com/2009/12/13/business/13drug.html.

18. J. Perz, and J. M. Ussher, "'The Horror of This Living Decay': Women's Negotiation and Resistance of Medical Discourses Around Menopause and Midlife," *Women's Studies International Forum,* vol. 31 (2008): 293–299.

19. For a review see B. Ayers, M. Forshaw, and M. S. Hunter, "The Impact of Attitudes Towards the Menopause on Women's Symptom Experience: A Systematic Review," *Maturitas* 65, no. 1 (2010): 28–36.

20. R. Bauld and Rhonda F. Brown, "Stress, Psychological Distress, Psychosocial Factors, Menopause Symptoms and Physical Health in Women," *Maturitas* 62, no. 2 (2009): 160–165.

21. H. E. Dillaway, "'Why Can't You Control This?' How Women's Interactions with Intimate Partners Define Menopause and Family," *Journal of Women and Aging* 20, no. 1–2 (2008): 47–64.

22. P. K. Mansfield, P. B. Koch, and G. Gierach, "Husbands' Support of Their Perimenopausal Wives," *Women and Health* 38, no. 3 (2003): 97–112.

23. R. L. Utz, "Like Mother, (Not) Like Daughter: The Social Construction of Menopause and Aging," *Journal of Aging Studies* 25, no. 2 (2011): 143–154.

24. A. Katz, "Observations and Advertising: Controversies in the Prescribing of Hormone Replacement Therapy," *Health Care for Women International* 24, no. 10 (2003): 927–939.

25. M. W. Matlin, "Women and Older Adulthood."

26. N. E. Avis and S. Crawford, "Cultural Differences in Symptoms and Attitudes Toward Menopause," *Menopause Management* 17, no. 3 (2008): 8–13.

27. M. Rotem, T. Kushnir, R. Levine, and M. Ehrenfeld, "A Psycho-Educational Program for Improving Women's Attitudes and Coping With Menopause Symptoms," *Journal of Obstetric, Gynecologic, and Neonatal Nursing* 34, no. 2 (2005): 233–240.

28. M. R. Soules, S. Sherman, E. Parrott, R. Rebar, N. Santoro, W. Utian, and N. Woods, "Executive Summary: Stages of Reproductive Aging Workshop (STRAW)," *Fertility and Sterility* 76, no. 5 (2001): 874–877; K. J. Carlson, S. A. Eisenstat, and T. D. Ziporyn. *The New Harvard Guide to Women's Health*. Vol. 1 (Cambridge, MA: Harvard University Press, 2004).

29. W. H. Utian, "Menopause-Related Definitions," *International Congress Series*, vol. 1266 (2004): 133–138.

30. A. L. Stanton et al., "Psychosocial Aspects of Selected Issues in Women's Reproductive Health."

31. M. R. Newhart, "Menopause Matters: The Implications of Menopause Research for Studies of Midlife Health," *Health Sociology Review* 22, no. 4 (2013): 365–376.

32. For a review see Z. A. Al-Safi and Nanette Santoro, "Menopausal Hormone Therapy and Menopausal Symptoms," *Fertility and Sterility* 101, no. 4 (2014): 905–907.

33. S. M. Bhattacharya and A. Jha, "A Comparison of Health-Related Quality of Life (HRQOL) After Natural and Surgical Menopause," *Maturitas* 66, no. 4 (2010): 431–434.

34. C. A. Morse, A. Smith, L. Dennerstein, A. Green, J. Hopper, and H. Burger, "The Treatment-Seeking Woman at Menopause," *Maturitas* 18, no. 3 (1994): 161–173.

35. M. K. Melby, M. Lock, and P. Kaufert, "Culture and Symptom Reporting at Menopause," *Human Reproduction Update* 11, no. 5 (2005): 495–512.

36. For a review see E. W. Freeman and K. Sherif, "Prevalence of Hot Flashes and Night Sweats Around the World: A Systematic Review," *Climacteric* 10, no. 3 (2007): 197–214.

37. L. Bairy, S. Adiga, P. Bhat, and R. Bhat, "Prevalence of Menopausal Symptoms and Quality of Life After Menopause in Women from South India," *Australian and New Zealand Journal of Obstetrics and Gynaecology* 49, no. 1 (2009): 106–109.

38. G. Richard-Davis and M. Wellons, "Racial and Ethnic Differences in the Physiology and Clinical Symptoms of Menopause," *Seminars in Reproductive Medicine* 31, no. 05 (2013): 380–386.

39. L. L. Sievert, *Menopause: A Biocultural Perspective* (New Brunswick, NJ: Rutgers University Press, 2006).

40. F. C. Baker, A. R. Willoughby, S. A. Sassoon, I. M. Colrain, and M. de Zambotti, "Insomnia in Women Approaching Menopause: Beyond Perception," *Psychoneuroendocrinology* 60 (2015): 96–104.

41. C. Storrs, "Exercise During Menopause Could Reduce Hot Flashes, Study Says," CNN .com, January, 27, 2016, http://www.cnn.com/2016/01/27/health/menopause-hot-flashes -exercise/.

42. L. Hauser, "Migraines and Perimenopause," *Nursing for Women's Health* 16, no. 3 (2012): 247–250.

43. V. T. Martin, "Migraine and the Menopausal Transition," *Neurological Sciences* 35, no. 1 (2014): 65–69.

44. S. Wang, J. Fuh, S. Lu, K. Juang, and P. Wang, "Migraine Prevalence During Meno-pausal Transition," *Headache: The Journal of Head and Face Pain* 43, no. 5 (2003): 470–478.

45. E. Loder, P. Rizzoli, and J. Golub, "Hormonal Management of Migraine Associated with Menses and the Menopause: A Clinical Review," *Headache: The Journal of Head and Face Pain* 47, no. 2 (2007): 329–340.

46. H. Buckler, "The Menopause Transition: Endocrine Changes and Clinical Symptoms," *British Menopause Society Journal* 11, no. 2 (2005): 61–65.

47. J. M. Ussher, "Menopause and the Ageing Body," 145.

48. S. L. Lewis, S. R. Dirksen, M. M. Heitkemper, and L. Bucher, "The Cardiovascular System," *Medical-Surgical Nursing: Assessment and Management of Clinical Problems* (Atlanta: Elsevier Health Sciences, 2013): 733.

49. K. Abernethy, "How the Menopause Affects the Cardiovascular Health of Women," *Primary Health Care* 18, no. 6 (2008): 41–47.

50. M. C. Carr, "The Emergence of the Metabolic Syndrome With Menopause," *The Journal of Clinical Endocrinology and Metabolism* 88, no. 6 (2003): 2404–2411.

51. Centers for Disease Control and Prevention, "Preventing Heart Disease: Healthy Living Habits." CDC (2015). Accessed October 02, 2016, http://www.cdc.gov/heart disease/healthy_living.htm.

52. Centers for Disease Control and Prevention, "Deaths: Final Data 2013," *National Vital Statistics Report* 64, no. 2, February 16, 2016, http://www.cdc.gov/nchs/data/nvsr/nvsr64 /nvsr64_02.pdf.

53. Ibid.

54. Ibid.

55. B. R. Hunt, S. Whitman, and M. S. Hurlbert, "Increasing Black: White Disparities in Breast Cancer Mortality in The 50 Largest Cities in the United States," *Cancer epide-miology* 38, no. 2 (2014): 118–123.

56. NIH Osteoporosis and Related Bone Diseases National Resource Center, "Bone Mass Measurement: What the Numbers Mean," June 2015, http://www.niams.nih.gov/health _info/bone/bone_health/bone_mass_measure.asp.

57. G. J. Tortora and S. R. Grabowski, *Principles of Anatomy and Physiology* (New York: Wiley, 2012): 926.

58. P. Ravn, M. L. Hetland, K. Overgaard, and C. Christiansen, "Premenopausal and Post-menopausal Changes in Bone Mineral Density of the Proximal Femur Measured by Dual-Energy X-Ray Absorptiometry," *Journal of Bone and Mineral Research* 9, no. 12 (1994): 1975–1980.

59. D. J. McLernon, J. J. Powell, R. Jugdaohsingh, and H. M. Macdonald, "Do Lifestyle Choices Explain the Effect of Alcohol on Bone Mineral Density in Women Around Menopause?" *The American Journal of Clinical Nutrition* 95, no. 5 (2012): 1261–1269.

60. For a review see K. Smith-DiJulio, N. F. Woods, and E. S. Mitchell, "Well-Being During the Menopausal Transition and Early Postmenopause: A Longitudinal Analysis." *Menopause* 15, no. 6 (2008): 1095–1102.

## Chapter 9: Aging Into One of the Happiest Times of Life

1. K. Heinemann, A. Ruebig, P. Potthoff, H. P. G. Schneider, F. Strelow, and L. A. J. Heinemann, "The Menopause Rating Scale (MRS) Scale: A Methodological Review," *Health and Quality of Life Outcomes* 2, no. 1 (2004): 1.

2. J. M. Ussher, "Menopause and the Ageing Body," 145; L. Hvas, "Menopausal Women's Positive Experience of Growing Older," *Maturitas* 54, no. 3 (2006): 245–251; L. Dennerstein, J. Randolph, J. Taffe, E. Dudley, and H. Burger, "Hormones, Mood, Sexuality, and the Menopausal Transition," *Fertility and Sterility* 77 (2002): 42–48.

3. A. L. Spencer and R. Bonnema, "Health Issues in Oral Contraception: Risks, Side Effects and Health Benefits," *Expert Review of Obstetrics and Gynecology* 6, no. 5 (2011): 551–557.

4. A. Darbonne, B. N. Uchino, and A. D. Ong, "What Mediates Links Between Age and Well-Being? A Test of Social Support and Interpersonal Conflict as Potential Interpersonal Pathways," *Journal of Happiness Studies* 14, no. 3 (2013): 951–63. doi:10.1007/s10902–012–9363–1.

5. M. W. Matlin, *The Psychology of Women*; J. Astbury, "Menopause," *Mental Health Aspects of Women's Reproductive Years: A Global Review of the Literature* (Geneva: WHO Press, 2009); N. E. Avis, "Depression During the Menopausal Transition," *Psychology of Women Quarterly* 27, no. 2 (2003): 91–100. doi:10.1111/1471–6402.00089

6. R. Worsley, R. J. Bell, P. Gartoulla, and S. R. Davis, "Low Use of Effective and Safe Therapies for Moderate to Severe Menopausal Symptoms: A Cross-Sectional Community Study of Australian Women," *Menopause* 23, no. 1 (2016): 11–17; A. C Guyton and J. E. Hall, "Female Physiology Before Pregnancy and Female Hormones," *Textbook of Medical Physiology*.

7. M. R. Newhart, "Menopause Matters: The Implications of Menopause Research for Studies of Midlife Health."

8. L. D. Butler and S. Nolen-Hoeksema, "Gender Differences in Responses to Depressed Mood in a College Sample," *Sex Roles* 30.5–6 (1994): 331–46.

9. S. Lyubomirsky, K. Layous, J. Chancellor, and S. K. Nelson, "Thinking About Rumination: The Scholarly Contributions and Intellectual Legacy of Susan Nolen-Hoeksema," *Annual Review of Clinical Psychology* 11 (2015): 1–22.

10. J. M. Ussher, "Are We Medicalizing Women's Misery? A Critical Review of Women's Higher Rates of Reported Depression," *Feminism and Psychology* 20, no. 1 (2010): 9–35; M. N. Lafrance, *Women and Depression: Recovery and Resistance* (London: Routledge, 2009).

11. J. H. Boyd, M. M. Weissman, W. D. Thompson, and J. K. Myers, "Screening for Depression in a Community Sample: Understanding the Discrepancies Between Depression Symptom and Diagnostic Scales," *Archives of General Psychiatry* 39, no. 10 (1982): 1195–1200.

12. National Addiction and HIV Data Archive Program, "National Survey on Drug Use and Health, 2013," November 23, 2015. doi.org/10.3886/ICPSR35509.v3.

13. Centers for Disease Control and Prevention, "National Health and Nutrition Survey Data 2007–2010," February 24, 2016, http://www.cdc.gov/nchs/nhanes/index.htm.

14. E. W. Freeman, "Associations of Depression with the Transition to Menopause," *Menopause* 17, no. 4 (2010): 823–27. doi:10.1097gme.0b013e3181db9f8b.

15. F. K. Judd, M. Hickey, and C. Bryant, "Depression and Midlife: Are We Overpathologising the Menopause?", *Journal of Affective Disorders* 136, no. 3 (2012): 199–211.

16. J. T. Bromberger, H. M. Kravitz, Y. F. Chang, J. M. Cyranowski, C. Brown, and K. A. Matthews, "Major Depression During and After the Menopausal Transition: Study of Women's Health Across the Nation (SWAN)," *Psychological Medicine* 41, no. 09 (2011): 1879–1888. doi:10.1017/s003329171100016x.

17. E. W. Freeman, M. D. Sammel, L. Liu, C. R. Gracia, D. B. Nelson, and L. Hollande, "Hormones and Menopausal Status as Predictors of Depression in Women in Transition to Menopause," *Archives of General Psychiatry* 61, no. 1 (2004): 62–70. doi:10.1001/archpsyc.61.1.62.

18. M. F. Morrison, E. W. Freeman, H. Lin, and M. D. Sammel, "Higher DHEA-S (Dehydroepiandrosterone Sulfate) Levels Are Associated with Depressive Symptoms During the Menopausal Transition: Results from the PENN Ovarian Aging Study," *Archives of Women's Mental Health* 14, no. 5 (2011): 375–382.

19. N. F. Woods, K. Smith-DiJulio, D. B. Percival, E. Y. Tao, A. Mariella, and E. S. Mitchell, "Depressed Mood During the Menopausal Transition and Early Postmenopause: Observations from the Seattle Midlife Women's Health Study." *Menopause* 15, no. 2 (2008): 223–232.

20. F. K. Judd et al., "Depression and Midlife: Are We Overpathologising the Menopause?"; P. Llaneza, M. P. García-Portilla, D. Llaneza-Suárez, B. Armott, and F. R. Pérez-López, "Depressive Disorders and the Menopause Transition," *Maturitas* 71, no. 2 (2012): 120–130

21. For a review see K. K. Vesco, E. M. Haney, L. Humphrey, R. Fu, and H. D. Nelson, "Influence of Menopause on Mood: A Systematic Review of Cohort Studies," *Climacteric* 10, no. 6 (2007): 448–465.

22. M. R. Newhart, "Menopause Matters: The Implications of Menopause Research for Studies of Midlife Health."

23. P. Llaneza et al., "Depressive Disorders and the Menopause Transition"; K. K. Vesco et al., "Influence of Menopause on Mood: A Systematic Review of Cohort Studies."

24. R. J. Boland, M. B. Keller, I. H. Gotlib, and C. L. Hammen, "Course and Outcome of Depression," *Handbook of Depression* 2 (2002): 23–43.

25. G. I. Metalsky and T. E. Joiner, "Vulnerability to Depressive Symptomatology: A Prospective Test of the Diathesis-Stress and Causal Mediation Components of the Hopelessness Theory of Depression," *Journal of Personality and Social Psychology* 63, no. 4 (1992): 667.

26. K. Smith-DiJulio et al., "Well-Being During the Menopausal Transition and Early Postmenopause: A Longitudinal Analysis"; E. W. Freeman, "Associations of Depression with the Transition to Menopause."

27. M.W. Matlin, *The Psychology of Women.*

28. S. S. Canetto, "Older Adulthood," *The Complete Guide to Mental Health for Women*, ed. L. Slater, J. H. Daniel, and A. E. Banks (Boston: Beacon Press, 2003).

29. J. T. Bromberger et al., "Major Depression During and After the Menopausal Transition: Study of Women's Health Across the Nation (SWAN)."

30. S. L. Brown and I.F. Lin, "The Gray Divorce Revolution: Rising Divorce Among Middle-Aged and Older Adults, 1990–2010," *The Journals of Gerontology Series B: Psychological Sciences and Social Sciences* 67, no. 6 (2012): 731–741. doi:10.1093/geronb/gbs089.

31. T. H. Holmes and R. H. Rahe, "The Social Readjustment Rating Scale," *Journal of Psychosomatic Research* 11, no. 2 (1967): 213–218.

32. P. R. Amato, "Research on Divorce: Continuing Trends and New Developments," *Journal of Marriage and Family* 72, no. 3 (2010): 650–666. doi:10.1111/j.1741–3737 .2010.00723.x.

33. R. Forste and T. B. Heaton, "The Divorce Generation," *Journal of Divorce and Remarriage* 41, no. 1–2 (2004): 95–114. doi:10.1300/j087v41n01_06.

34. L. Dennerstein et al., "Hormones, Mood, Sexuality, and the Menopausal Transition," *Fertility and Sterility* 77 (2002): 42–48.

35. L. Liu, Z. Gou, and J. Zuo, "Social Support Mediates Loneliness and Depression in Elderly People." *Journal of Health Psychology* (2014): 1359105314536941.

36. S. Cohen, L. G. Underwood, and B. H. Gottlieb, *Social Support Measurement and Intervention: A Guide for Health and Social Scientists* (Oxford: Oxford University Press, 2000).

37. For a review see K. Smith-DiJulio et al., "Well-Being During the Menopausal Transition and Early Postmenopause: A Longitudinal Analysis."

## Chapter 10: Be Afraid of the Menopausal Profit Monster

1. A. Spake, "The Menopausal Marketplace," *US News & World Report*, November 18, 2002: 1–6.

2. B. Seaman, *The Greatest Experiment Ever Performed on Women.*

3. R. Moynihan and A. Cassels, "Working with Celebrities: Menopause," *Selling Sickness: How the Worlds' Biggest Pharmaceutical Companies Are Turning Us All into Patients* (New York: Nation Books, 2005).

4. B. Seaman, *The Greatest Experiment Ever Performed on Women.*

5. H. K. Ziel, and W. D. Finkle, "Increased Risk of Endometrial Carcinoma Among Users of Conjugated Estrogens," *New England Journal of Medicine* 293, no. 23 (1975): 1167-1170.

6. S. Coney, *The Menopause Industry: How the Medical Establishment Exploits Women*, (Alameda, CA: Hunter House, 1994).

7. R. Hoover, L. A. Gray, P. Cole, and B. Macmahon, "Menopausal Estrogens and Breast Cancer," *New England Journal of Medicine* 295, no. 8 (1976): 401–05. doi:10.1056/nejm 197608192950801.

8. Boston Collaborative Drug Surveillance Program, "Surgically Confirmed Gallbladder Disease, Venous Thromboembolism, and Breast Tumors in Relation to Postmenopausal Estrogen Therapy," *New England Journal of Medicine* 290, no. 1 (1974): 15–29. doi: 10.1056/nejm197401032900104.

9.  P. Kaufert and S. McKinlay, "Estrogen-Replacement Therapy: The Production of Medical Knowledge and the Emergence of Policy," *Women, Health, and Healing* ed. E. Lewin and V. Olesen (London: Tavistock Press, 2005): 113–38.

10. Ibid.

11. S. Coney, *The Menopause Industry.*

12. B. Seaman, *The Greatest Experiment Ever Performed on Women.*

13. H. K. Genant, "Quantitative Computed Tomography of Vertebral Spongiosa: A Sensitive Method for Detecting Early Bone Loss After Oophorectomy," *Annals of Internal Medicine* 97, no. 5 (1982): 699–705. doi:10.7326/0003–4819–97–5-699.

14. B. Seaman, *The Greatest Experiment Ever Performed on Women.*

15. N. C. Wright, A. C. Looker, K. G. Saag, J. R. Curtis, E. S. Delzell, S. Randall, and B. Dawson-Hughes, "The Recent Prevalence of Osteoporosis and Low Bone Mass in the United States Based on Bone Mineral Density at the Femoral Neck or Lumbar Spine," *Journal of Bone and Mineral Research* 29, no. 11 (2014): 2520–2526.

16. S. E. Sattui, and K. G. Saag, "Fracture Mortality: Associations with Epidemiology and Osteoporosis Treatment," *Nature Reviews Endocrinology* 10, no. 10 (2014): 592–602. doi:10.1038/nrendo.2014.125.

17. S. Coney, *The Menopause Industry.*

18. Advertisement for Estraderm, *The Journal of Clinical Medicine, Modern Medicine* 38 (1995): 156.

19. Harvard Health Publications, "Estrogen and Your Arteries," *Harvard Women's Health Watch* (1995): 6.

20. M. J. Naughton, A. S. Jones, and S. A. Shumaker, "When Practices, Promises, Profits, and Policies Outpace Hard Evidence: The Post-Menopausal Hormone Debate," *Journal of Social Issues* 61, no. 1 (2005): 159–179. doi:10.1111/j.0022–4537.2005.00399.x.

21. Ibid.

22. S. Hulley, "Randomized Trial of Estrogen Plus Progestin for Secondary Prevention of Coronary Heart Disease in Postmenopausal Women." *Journal of the American Medical Association* 280, no. 7 (1998): 605–13. doi:10.1001/jama.280.7.605.

23. R. Moynihan and A. Cassels, "Working with Celebrities: Menopause," *Selling Sickness.*

24. Ibid.

25. P. Cram, A. M. Fendrick, J. Inadomi, M. E. Cowen, D. Carpenter, and S. Vijan, "The Impact of a Celebrity Promotional Campaign on the Use of Colon Cancer Screening," *Archives of Internal Medicine* 163, no. 13 (July 14, 2003): 1601. doi:10.1001/archinte .163.13.1601.

26. M. L. Palley, "Rethinking a Women's Health Care Agenda in the United States," *The Politics of Women's Health Care in the US*, ed. H. A. Palley (New York: Palgrave Pivot, 2014).

27. Women's Health Initiative, "Design of the Women's Health Initiative Clinical Trial and Observational Study," *Controlled Clinical Trials* 19, no. 1 (1998): 61–109.

28. Writing Group for the Women's Health Initiative Investigators, "Risks and Benefits of Estrogen Plus Progestin in Healthy Postmenopausal Women: Principal Results from the Women's Health Initiative Randomized Controlled Trial," *JAMA* 288, no. 3 (2002): 321–333. doi:10.1001/jama.288.3.321.

29. M. J. Naughton et al., "When Practices, Promises, Profits, and Policies Outpace Hard Evidence: The Post-Menopausal Hormone Debate."

30. S. W. Junod, "FDA and Clinical Drug Trials: A Short History," US Food and Drug Administration, April 11, 2016, www.fda.gov/aboutFDA/WhatWeDo/History/Overviews/ucm304485.htm.

31. M. J. Naughton et al., "When Practices, Promises, Profits, and Policies Outpace Hard Evidence: The Post-Menopausal Hormone Debate."

32. S. Hensley, "Wyeth Stock Slides as Study Casts Shadow on Medicines." *Wall Street Journal*, July 10, 2002, http://www.wsj.com/articlesSB1026247768607338960.

33. Ibid.; S. Hensley and P. Landers, "Drug Companies Report Pain," *Wall Street Journal*, October 23, 2003, http://www.wsj.com/articles/SB106649716764745700.

34. H. Brody, "The Company We Keep: Why Physicians Should Refuse to See Pharmaceutical Representatives," *Annuls of Family Medicine* (2005): 82–85. doi:10.1370/afm.259.

35. S. Sah, "Conflicts of Interest and Your Physician: Psychological Processes That Cause Unexpected Changes in Behavior," *The Journal of Law, Medicine and Ethics* 40, no. 3 (2012): 482–487. doi:10.1111/j.1748–720x.2012.00680.x.

36. T. Bodenheimer, "Uneasy Alliance—Clinical Investigators and the Pharmaceutical Industry," *New England Journal of Medicine* 342, no. 20 (May 18, 2000): 1539–544. doi:10.1056/nejm200005183422024.

37. A. Fugh-Berman, C. P. Mcdonald, A. M. Bell, E. C. Bethards, and A. R. Scialli, "Promotional Tone in Reviews of Menopausal Hormone Therapy After the Women's Health Initiative: An Analysis of Published Articles," *PLOS Medicine* 8, no. 3 (March 15, 2011). doi:10.1371/journal.pmed.1000425.

38. Ibid.

39. "Understanding Menopause Treatment" *WebMD*, accessed September 21, 2016, http://www.webmd.com/menopause/guide/understanding-menopause-treatment.

40. US Food and Drug Administration, "Bio-Identicals: Sorting Myths from Facts," April 8, 2008, http://www.fda.gov/ForConsumers/ConsumerUpdates/ucm049311.htm.

41. J. Conaway, "Bioidentical Hormones: An Evidence-Based Review for Primary Care Providers," *The Journal of the American Osteopathic Association* 111, no. 3 (2011): 153–64.

42. Pinkerton, J. V., and N. Santoro, "Compounded Bioidentical Hormone Therapy: Identifying Use Trends and Knowledge Gaps Among US Women," *Menopause* 22, no. 9 (2015): 926. doi:10.1097/gme.0000000000000420.

43. *For a review see* J. Conaway, "Bioidentical Hormones: An Evidence-Based Review for Primary Care Providers."

44. E. Schwartz, "Letter to Suzanne Somers," October 15, 2006, http://drerika.typepad.com/notepad/2006/10/letter_to_suzan.html.

# Chapter 11: How Lies Persist and What We Lose by Believing Them

1. J. C. Chrisler et al., "The PMS Illusion."

2. S. L. Bem, *Lenses of Gender: Transforming the Debate on Sexual Inequality* (New Haven, CT: Yale University Press, 1993).

3. K. Bussey, and A. Bandura, "Social Cognitive Theory of Gender Development and Differentiation," *Psychological Review* 106, no. 4 (1999): 676–713. doi:10.1037//0033–295 x.106.4.676.

4. J. S. Hyde, "Gender Similarities and Differences," *Annual Review of Psychology* 65, no. 1 (2014): 373–98. doi:10.1146/annurev-psych-010213–115057.

5. M. W. Matlin, "Infancy and Childhood," *The Psychology of Women*.

6. Ibid.

7. J. E.O. Blakemore, "Children's Beliefs about Violating Gender Norms: Boys Shouldn't Look like Girls and Girls Shouldn't Act like Boys," *Sex Roles* 56 (2003): 393–421. doi:10.1023/A:1023574427720.

8. M. S. Kimmel, "Bros Before Hos: The Guy Code," *Guyland: The Perilous World Where Boys Become Men* (New York: Harper, 2008).

9. E. Wilbur, "Boomer No Fan of Paternity Leave," *Boston.com*, April 15, 2014, http://archive.boston.com/sports/baseball/2014/04/03/have-section-boomer-esiason-fan-paternity-leave/CFjcunBotpj4Hb4kxi8C4O/story.html.

10. J. S. Hyde, "Gender Similarities and Differences," *Annual Review of Psychology* 65, no. 1 (2014): 373–98. doi:10.1146/annurev-psych-010213–115057.

11. J. B. Becker and M. Hu, "Sex Differences in Drug Abuse," *Frontiers in Neuroendocrinology* 29, no. 1 (2008): 36–47. doi:10.1016/j.yfrne.2007.07.003.

12. R. Rosenthal, "Interpersonal Expectations: Some Antecedents and Some Consequences," *Interpersonal Expectations: Theory, Research, and Applications,* ed. P. D Blank (Cambridge: Cambridge University Press, 1993): 3–24.

13. C. M. Steele, S. J. Spencer, and J. Aronson, "Contending with Group Image: The Psychology of Stereotype and Social Identity Threat," *Advances in Experimental Social Psychology* 34, (2002): 379–440. doi:10.1016/s0065–2601(02)80009–0.

14. J. Flanagan, "Gender and the Workplace: The Impact of Stereotype Threat on Self-Assessment of Management Skills of Female Business Students," *Advancing Women in Leadership* 35 (2015): 166–71.

15. E. C. Pinel and Nicole Paulin, "Stigma Consciousness at Work," *Basic and Applied Social Psychology* 27, no. 4 (2005): 345–52. doi:10.1207/s15324834basp2704_7.

16. N. D. Spector, W. Cull, S. R. Daniels, J. Gilhooly, J. Hall, I. Horn, S. G. Marshall, D. J. Schumacher, T. C. Sectish, and B. F. Stanton. "Gender and Generational Influences on the Pediatric Workforce and Practice," *Pediatrics* 133, no. 6 (May 2014): 1112-121. doi:10.1542/peds.2013-3016.

17. C. Peckam, "Medscape Physician Compensation Report 2015," *Medscape Physician Compensation Report 2015,* accessed October 01, 2016, http://www.medscape.com/features/slideshow/compensation/2015/public/overview#page=3.

18. B. Major and Laurie T. O'Brien, "The Social Psychology of Stigma," *Annual Review of Psychology* 56, no. 1 (2005): 393–421. doi:10.1146/annurev.psych.56.091103.070137.

19. J. C. Blickenstaff, "Women and Science Careers: Leaky Pipeline or Gender Filter?" *Gender and Education* 17, no. 4 (2005): 369–86. doi:10.1080/09540250500145072.

20. T. N. Greenstein, "Husbands' Participation in Domestic Labor: Interactive Effects of Wives' and Husbands' Gender Ideologies," *Journal of Marriage and the Family* 58, no. 3 (1996): 585–95. doi:10.2307/353719.

21. R. Gaunt, "Biological Essentialism, Gender Ideologies, and Role Attitudes: What Determines Parents' Involvement in Child Care," *Sex Roles* 55, no. 7–8 (2006): 523–33. doi:10.1007/s11199–006–9105–0.

22. L. C. Sayer and S. M. Bianchi, "Women's Economic Independence and the Probability of Divorce: A Review and Reexamination," *Journal of Family Issues* 21, no. 7 (2000): 906–43. doi:10.1177/019251300021007005.

23. For a review see M. P. Atkinson, T. N. Greenstein, and M. M. Lang, "For Women, Breadwinning Can Be Dangerous: Gendered Resource Theory and Wife Abuse," *Journal of Marriage and Family* 67, no. 5 (2005): 1–22. doi:10.1111/j.1741–3737.2005 .00206.x.

24. P. Voydanoff, *Work, Family, and Community: Exploring Interconnections* (Mahwah, NJ: Lawrence Erlbaum Associates, 2007).

25. P. R. Amato and A. Booth, "Changes in Gender Role Attitudes and Perceived Marital Quality," *American Sociological Review* 60, no. 1 (1995): 58–66. doi:10.2307/2096345.

26. K. T. Bui, B. H. Raven, and J. Schwartzwald, "Influence Strategies in Dating Relationships: The Effects of Relationship Satisfaction, Gender, and Perspective," *Journal of Social Behavior and Personality* 9, no. 3 (1994): 429–42.

27. J. Schwarzwald, M. Koslowsky, and E. B. Izhak-Nir, "Gender Role Ideology as a Moderator of the Relationship Between Social Power Tactics and Marital Satisfaction," *Sex Roles* 59, no. 9–10 (2008): 657–69. doi:10.1007/s11199–008–9454-y.

28. Center for American Women in Politics, "Women in State Legislatures 2016," accessed April 20, 2016, http://www.cawp.rutgers.edu/women-state-legislature-2016.

29. L. Kent, "Number of Women Leaders Around the World Has Grown, But They're Still a Small Group," *PewResearchCenter*, July 30, 2015, http://www.pewresearch.org/fact -tank/2015/07/30/about-one-in-ten-of-todays-world-leaders-are-women/

30. A. H. Eagly, *Sex Differences in Social Behavior: A Social-role Interpretation* (Hillsdale, NJ: L. Erlbaum Associates, 1987).

31. C. H. Tinsley, S. I. Cheldelin, A. K. Schneider, and E. T. Amanatullah, "Negotiating Your Public Identity: Women's Path to Power," *Rethinking Negotiation Teaching: Innovations For Context And Culture*, ed. C. Honeyman, J. Coben, and G. De Palo (Saint Paul, MN: DRI Press, 2009).

32. A. E. Kornblut, *Notes from the Cracked Ceiling: Hillary Clinton, Sarah Palin, and What It Will Take for a Woman to Win* (New York: Crown Publishers, 2009).

33. M. Reston, "Hillary Clinton's Gender Politics," *CNN.com*, January 5, 2015, http://www .cnn.com/2015/01/05/politics/hillary-clinton-gender/.

34. K. Dion, E. Berscheid, and E. Walster, "What Is Beautiful Is Good," *Journal of Personality and Social Psychology* 24, no. 3 (1972): 285–90. doi:10.1037/h0033731.

35. C. L. Toma and J. T. Hancock, "Looks and Lies: The Role of Physical Attractiveness in Online Dating Self-Presentation and Deception," *Communication Research* 37, no. 3 (2010): 335–51. doi:10.1177/0093650209356437.

36. S. K. Johnson, K. E. Podratz, R. L. Dipboye, and E. Gibbons, "Physical Attractiveness Biases in Ratings of Employment Suitability: Tracking Down the 'Beauty Is Beastly' Effect," *The Journal of Social Psychology* 150, no. 3 (2010): 301–18. doi: 10.1080/00224540903365414.

37. A. E. Kornblut, *Notes from the Cracked Ceiling.*

38. P. Cheng, "Palin Magazine Cover Draws Ire from New Yorkers," *NBC*, November 17, 2009, http://www.nbcnewyork.com/news/Palin-Magazine-Cover-Draws-Ire-70339082.html.

39. S. Muller, "Sexist 'KFC' Hillary Clinton Buttons at GOP Event," *MSNBC.com*, October 8, 2013, http://www.msnbc.com/the-last-word/sexist-anti-clinton-buttons-gop-event.

## Conclusion: Protecting the Powerful Reality of Women

1. S. Malo, "In US First, New York City Making Tampons Free in Schools," *Thomas Reuters Foundation*, June 22, 2016, http://news.trust.org/item/20160622190703-fymsf.

2. A. Jones, "The Fight against Period Shaming Is Going Mainstream," *Newsweek*. April 20, 2016, http://www.newsweek.com/2016/04/29/womens-periods-menstruation-tampons-pads-449833.html.

3. G. Steinem, "If Men Could Menstruate," *Ms. Magazine*, October 1978.

4. D. A. Smith, D. Vivian, and K. D. O'Leary, "Longitudinal Prediction of Marital Discord from Premarital Expressions of Affect," *Journal of Consulting and Clinical Psychology* 58, no. 6 (1990): 790–98. doi:10.1037//0022–006x.58.6.790.

5. M. Epstein and L. M. Ward "'Always Use Protection': Communication Boys Receive About Sex From Parents, Peers, and the Media," *Journal of Youth and Adolescence* 37, no. 2 (2008): 113–26. doi:10.1007/s10964–007 9187–1.

6. J. M. Wood, P. B. Koch, and P. K. Mansfield, "Is My Period Normal? How College-Aged Women Determine the Normality or Abnormality of Their Menstrual Cycles," *Women and Health* 46, no. 1 (2007): 41–56. doi:10.1300/j013v46n01_04.

7. L. S. Dumas, *Talking with Kids about Tough Issues* (Menlo Park, CA: Henry J. Kaiser Family Foundation, 1996).

8. J. B. Gillooly, "Making Menarche Positive and Powerful for Both Mother and Daughter," *Women and Therapy* 27, no. 3–4 (2004): 23–35. doi:10.1300/j015v27n03_03.

9. Ibid.

10. M. Epstein et al., "'Always Use Protection': Communication Boys Receive About Sex From Parents, Peers, and the Media."

11. K. R. Allen, C. E. Kaestle, and A. E. Goldberg, "More Than Just a Punctuation Mark: How Boys and Young Men Learn About Menstruation," *Journal of Family Issues* 32, no. 2 (2010): 129–56. doi:10.1177/0192513x10371609.

12. J. Rivas, "Half of Young People Believe Gender Isn't Limited to Male and Female," *Fusion*, February 3, 2015, http://fusion.net/story/42216/half-of-young-people-believe-gender-isnt-limited-to-male-and-female/.

13. D. S. Pedulla and S. Thebaud, "Can We Finish the Revolution? Gender, Work-Family Ideals, and Institutional Constraint," *American Sociological Review* 80, no. 1 (2015): 116–39. doi:10.1177/0003122414564008.

## Appendix I: Women's Hormones: An Overview

1. K. J. Carlson, S. A. Eisenstat, and T. D. Ziporyn, *The New Harvard Guide to Women's Health* (Cambridge, MA: Harvard University Press, 2004).

2. M. S. Rosenthal, *The Gynecological Sourcebook* (New York: McGraw-Hill, 2003).

# Appendix II: Ways to Spot Junk Science

1.  M. W. Matlin, "The Health Care and Health Status of Women," *The Psychology of Women*, 356–57.

2.  American Heart Association, "Heart Attack Symptoms in Women," July 2015, accessed October 01, 2016, http://www.heart.org/HEARTORG/Conditions/HeartAttack/WarningSignsofaHeartAttack/Heart-Attack-Symptoms-in-Women_UCM_436448_Article.jsp#.V3_feJMrJn4.

3.  J. L. Cox, J. M. Holden, and R. Sagovsky, "Detection of Postnatal Depression: Development of the 10-Item Edinburgh Postnatal Depression Scale," *The British Journal of Psychiatry* 150, no. 6 (June 1987): 782–86. doi:10.1192/bjp.150.6.782.

4.  S. Hearold, "A Synthesis of 1043 Effects of Television on Social Behavior," *Public Communications and Behavior*, ed. G. Comstock (New York: Academic Press, 1986): 65–133.

5.  B. Major, C. Cozzarelli, M. L. Cooper, J. Zubek, C. Richards, M. Wilhite, and R. H. Gramzow, "Psychological Responses of Women After First-Trimester Abortion," *Archives of General Psychiatry* 57, no. 8 (2000): 777–84. doi:10.1001/archpsyc.57.8.777; D. I. Rees and J. J. Sabia, "The Relationship Between Abortion and Depression: New Evidence from the Fragile Families and Child Wellbeing Study," *Medical Science Monitor* 13, no. 10 (2007): 430–36. doi:10.12659/msm.502357.

6.  N. Russo, "Understanding Emotional Responses after Abortion," *Lectures on the Psychology of Women*, ed. J. C. Chrisler, C. Golden, and P. D. Rozee (New York: McGraw-Hill, 2008): 172–89.

7.  P. Offit, "Alternative Medicines Are Popular, But Do Any of Them Really Work?" *The Washington Post*, November 12, 2013, https://www.washingtonpost.com/national/health-science/alternative-medicines-are-popular-but-do-any-of-them-really-work/2013/11/11/067f9272-004f-11e3-9711-3708310f6f4d_story.html.

8.  S. Shields, "Functionalism, Darwinism, and the Psychology of Women," *American Psychologist* 30, no. 7 (1975): 739–54. doi:10.1037/h0076948.

9.  J. R. Speakman, and S. E. Mitchell, "Caloric Restriction," *Molecular Aspects of Medicine* 32, no. 3 (2011): 159–221. doi:10.1016/j.mam.2011.07.001.

10. J. A. Mattison, G. S. Roth, T. M. Beasley, E. M. Tilmont, A. M. Handy, R. L. Herbert, D. L. Longo, D. B. Allison, J. E. Young, M. Bryant, D. Barnard, W. F. Ward, W. Qi, D. K. Ingram, and R. De Cabo, "Impact of Caloric Restriction on Health and Survival in Rhesus Monkeys from the NIA Study," *Nature* 489, no. 7415 (2012): 318–21. doi:10.1038/nature11432.

11. J. R. Speakman and S. E. Mitchell, "Caloric Restriction," *Molecular Aspects of Medicine* 32, no. 3 (2011): 159–221. doi:10.1016/j.mam.2011.07.001.

**Robyn Stein DeLuca, PhD,** is a research assistant professor in the department of psychology at Stony Brook University, and was a core faculty member of the women's and gender studies program for fifteen years. She has taught a multitude of courses on health, gender, and reproduction, and her research on postpartum depression and childbirth satisfaction has been published in scholarly psychology journals. Her TEDx Talk "The Good News About PMS" has had over one million views and has been translated into twenty-two languages.

# Index

bioidentical hormones, 141–143

biological essentialism, 149–150, 161

bipolar disorder, 98

birth-control pills, 40

body image: menopause and, 105–106; pregnancy and, 58

bone density, 118, 134–135, 139

breast cancer, 117–118, 139

breastfeeding, and medication use, 96–97

*British Medical Journal,* 24

## C

caffeine withdrawal, 37

California Milk Processor Board ad campaign, 18

caloric restriction, 187

cancer risks, 117, 132–133, 139

cardiovascular disease, 117

career choices, 155–157

categorizations, 167

CES-D scale, 125, 126

chasteberry, 41

Chesler, Phyllis, 35

childbirth: postpartum disorders after, 79–90, 93–99; social/ communal support following, 103–104. *See also* motherhood

childcare stress, 48, 95

children: raising to resist the hormone myth, 171–173; risks of postpartum disorders to, 100–101

China, PMS research in, 30

Chodorow, Nancy, 151

cholesterol levels, 117

clinics for PMS and PMDD treatment, 42

Clinton, Hillary, 159–160, 161

cognitive functioning: menstrual cycle and, 9–10; pregnancy and, 53–55, 59–61

comedians, PMS jokes told by, 16

competence conundrum, 159–160

compounding pharmacies, 142

conflict resolution, 157–158

control groups, 28–29, 182–183

Couric, Katie, 88, 137–138

Cox, Courtney, 81

cult of true womanhood, 44

culture: attitudes about menopause related to, 112; PMS as unique to Western, 30; postpartum depression related to, 96

## D

*Daily Mail,* 83

*Daily Telegraph,* 59

Dalton, Katharina, 23–24, 29, 46

dementia, 135–136, 139

demographics used in studies, 180

Department of Health and Human Services (HHS), 184

depression: menopausal women and, 123–127; psychological categorization of, 124–125; risk related to personal history of, 128; studies on hormones and, 126–127. *See also* postpartum depression

Deschanel, Zooey, 16

*Diagnostic and Statistical Manual of Mental Disorders:* diagnosing mental disorders using, 33–34; discussions behind revisions to,

35–37; transformation of PMS in, 30–32

diagnostic criteria: *DSM* transformation of PMS, 30–32; lack of standardization in PMS, 27–28

dietary concerns in pregnancy, 69–70

dietary supplements: PMS treatments using, 41; profit motive in research on, 185–186

divorce, empty-nest, 129–130

docile ideal, 44–45

domesticity, cult of, 44

Down syndrome, 71

drugs. *See* medications

## E

early menopause transition, 114

ectopic pregnancy, 67

Edinburgh Postnatal Depression Scale (EPDS), 181

educated consumer of research, 188

Eli Lilly and Company, 38–39

emotions: expressing angry thoughts and, 50–51; need for venting, 49–50; pregnancy and, 55–56, 57, 63

employed women. *See* working women

employment discrimination, 75–76

empty-nest divorces, 129–130

Ephron, Nora, 128

Equal Employment Opportunity Commission (EEOC), 75–76

equal status backlash, 51–52

Esiason, Boomer, 153

Estraderm patch, 135

estrogen, 177–178; heart disease and, 135; menopausal women and, 114, 116; pregnancy and production of, 56. *See also* hormone therapy

European-American women, 112, 117, 118

evening primrose oil, 41

## F

false uniqueness, 146

Falwell, Jerry, 47

*Feminine Forever* (Wilson), 108, 109, 132

feminism, 47

financial insecurity, 129

flu vaccine, 70

fluoxetine, 38

follicle stimulating hormone (FSH), 114, 177

Frank, Robert, 23, 45

## G

gender polarization, 149, 161

gender stereotypes, 17, 150–161; career choices and, 155–157; internal policing of, 153–154; marriage relationship and, 157–159; media outrage and, 153; parents and, 151–152; peers and, 152–153; politics and, 159–161; workplace and, 154–157

generosity, 170–171

Gilman, Charlotte Perkins, 45

ginko biloba, 185–186

*Girlfriends' Guide to Pregnancy, The* (Iovine), 55–56

illusory optimism, 145–146

*I'm Too Young for This* (Somers), 142

*Independent Conservative* website, 88–89

India, PMS research in, 30

information sources, 180

insomnia, 116

## J

joyful symptoms, 30

junk vs. good science, 179–188

## K

Kelly, Megyn, 13, 171

Kimmel, Michael, 152–153

## L

laboratory studies, 183

late luteal premenstrual dysphoric disorder (LLPDD), 36

late menopause transition, 114

Latina/Hispanic women, 112, 117

lesbian relationships, 51–52

Liddy, G. Gordon, 12–13

longevity study, 187

luteinizing hormone (LH), 114, 177

## M

major depression, 124

marital bargain, 107

marriage: conflict resolution in, 157–158; gender stereotypes in, 157–159; menopause and, 107–108, 111; postpartum depression and, 95, 101–103; pregnancy and, 58–59

May, Shannon, 89

Mayo Clinic, 81, 83

media: Andrea Yates case in, 87–89, 90; baby brain reported in, 59, 61–62; descriptions of menstruation by, 7; gender stereotypes in, 153; good vs. junk science in, 179–188; hormone myth reinforced in, 4; PMS themes in, 14–16; postpartum depression in, 82–84

medicalization of pregnancy, 66–67

medications: over-the-counter, 41–42; postpartum depression, 96–97; postpartum psychosis, 97; rebranded for PMDD, 38–40

memory: pregnancy and, 60–61. *See also* cognitive functioning

men: books about PMS for, 15; gender stereotypes and, 150, 152, 154; menstrual accusation between, 9

menopause, 105–144; aging-related challenges in, 127–130; biological changes during, 113–114; changing the perception of, 166; depression related to, 123–127; exposure to positive views about, 112–113; femininity maintenance and, 107–108; generational norms related to, 111–112; historical acknowledgment of, 106–107; hormone myth related to, 148–149; hormone replacement therapy for, 108–110, 131–144;

media depiction of, 105, 106; mythic attitudes about, 110–113; physical symptoms related to, 114–119; positive aspects of, 121–123; racial and cultural views about, 112; social support for women in, 130; spousal responses to, 111

menstrual accusation, 8–9

menstrual leave policies, 13

menstruation: career advancement and, 12–13; changing the perception of, 164–165; cognitive functioning and, 9–10; educating children about, 172, 173; joyful symptoms around, 30; menopause as end of, 121–122; negative attitudes about, 7–8, 10–13; PMS myth related to, 43; popular accusation related to, 8–9; puberty and start of, 19, 20–21; sexual attitudes related to, 12; societal stigmatization of, 8; teaching girls about, 172; themes about PMS and, 14–19

mental disorders: diagnosing in women, 33–35; effects of being diagnosed with, 32–33; PMS and biomedical model of, 25; postpartum psychosis and, 85–86; profit motive related to, 37–38

mental health: early maturing girls and, 20–21; pregnancy and, 56–57, 63; puberty/adolescence and, 19–20

*Miami Herald*, 84

Middleton, Kate, 79

Midol, 41

midwifery model, 72–73

migraine headaches, 116

mild depression, 125

Miltown, 34

Mirren, Helen, 128

*Modern Family*, 54

motherhood: day-to-day reality of, 48; living up to the mystique of, 91–92; postpartum disorders in, 79–87; risks of delaying, 77; social support for, 103–104. *See also* parenting

motherhood penalty, 77

Murphy, Daniel, 153

# N

National Association of Social Workers (NASW), 36

National Institutes of Health (NIH), 138, 184

National Organization of Women (NOW), 88

*National Review*, 88

Neeson, Liam, 128

*New England Journal of Medicine*, 132

*New Girl, The*, 16

*New York Times*, 14, 83

night sweats, 116

nocebo effect, 10–11

Northrup, Christiane, 110, 143

# O

objectification of women, 11–12

*Once a Month* (Dalton), 24

oophorectomy, 134

oral contraceptives, 40

osteoporosis, 118, 134–135, 139
*Our Bodies, Ourselves,* 110
over-the-counter drugs, 41–42
Oz, Mehmet, 14

# P

Palin, Sarah, 161
Paltrow, Gwyneth, 94
Panettiere, Hayden, 83
parenting: gender stereotypes
    reinforced through, 151–152;
    hormone myth countered by,
    171–173. *See also* motherhood
*Parents* magazine, 81, 82
Paxil, 40
peers: gender stereotypes
    reinforced by, 152–153;
    learning about menstruation
    from, 173
Penn Ovarian Aging Study
    (POAS), 126
perimenopause, 114
periods. *See* menstruation
pharmaceutical companies:
    hormone myth reinforced by, 4;
    physicians and, 140–141;
    pursuit of profit by, 38, 131–
    132, 140–141, 184; rebranding
    of Prozac for PMDD by, 38–40
physicians: hormone myth
    reinforced by, 4; medicalization
    of pregnancy by, 66–67;
    pharmaceutical companies and,
    140–141
*Physician's Desk Reference,* 33
placebo effect, 10
placenta previa, 67
"Playing God On No Sleep"
    (Quindlen), 87–88

PMDD (premenstrual dysphoric
    disorder): clinics for PMS and,
    42; common treatments for, 33,
    39–40; *DSM* guidelines for,
    30–32; effects of being
    diagnosed with, 32–33;
    hormone therapy for, 40;
    rebranding of Prozac for, 38–39
PMS (premenstrual syndrome),
    13–19; applied definition of, 25;
    clinics for treatment of, 42;
    debate about including in
    *DSM,* 35–36; diagnostic
    transformation to PMDD,
    30–32; framing requests for
    help using, 49; hormone
    therapy for, 33, 40; jokes,
    tweets, and stereotypes about,
    16–17; media and literary bias
    about, 14–16; moodiness myth
    around, 146–147; origin and
    perpetuation of concept of,
    23–25; over-the-counter
    treatments for, 41–42; personal
    responsibility myth about,
    18–19; problems with research
    on, 27–30; profit motive related
    to, 37–38; symptoms attributed
    to, 25–27; used as excuse by
    women, 52; working women
    and, 45–46
politics, 159–161; attractiveness
    conundrum in, 160–161;
    competence conundrum in,
    159–160
postmenopause, 114
postpartum blues, 82, 93, 99
postpartum depression, 79–84,
    93–97; assumptions vs. realities

**You've read the book—now spread the word!**

Download **The Hormone Myth Reading Group Guide** at

newharbinger.com/hormoneguide

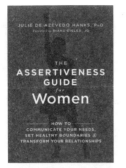
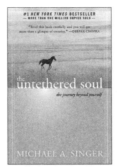
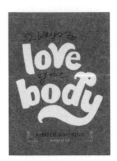
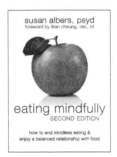
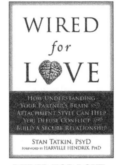
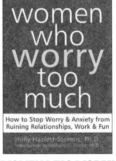